Annales Nestlé

Mother and Child Nutrition

Editor
Maria Makrides, Adelaide

S. Karger
Medical and Scientific Publishers
Basel · Freiburg · Paris ·
London · New York ·
Bangalore · Bangkok · Shanghai ·
Singapore · Tokyo · Sydney

KARGER

Nestlé
Nutrition
Institute

S. Karger
Medical and Scientific Publishers
Basel • Freiburg • Paris • London
New York • Bangalore • Bangkok
Shanghai • Singapore • Tokyo • Sydney

Disclaimer
Nestlé Nutrition-Nestec Ltd./S. Karger AG cannot be held responsible for errors or omissions, or for any consequences arising from the use of the information contained herein.

Drug Dosage
The authors and the publisher have exerted every effort to ensure that drug selection and dosage set forth in this text are in accord with current recommendations and practice at the time of publication. However, in view of ongoing research, changes in government regulations, and the constant flow of information relating to drug therapy and drug reactions, the reader is urged to check the package insert for each drug for any change in indications and dosage and for added warnings and precautions. This is particularly important when the recommended agent is a new and/or infrequently employed drug.

P.O. Box, CH–4009 Basel (Switzerland)
Printed in Switzerland on acid-free paper by
Reinhardt Druck, Basel (Switzerland)
ISBN 978–3–8055–9507–0
e-ISBN 978–3–8055–9508–7

KARGER

Fax +41 61 306 12 34
E-Mail karger@karger.ch
www.karger.com

Vol. 68, No. 1, 2010

Annales Nestlé

Contents

KARGER

Fax +41 61 306 12 34
E-Mail karger@karger.ch
www.karger.com

Access to full text and tables of contents,
including tentative ones for forthcoming issues:
www.karger.com/ane_issues

Policy Statement

The Nestlé Nutrition Institute was created to provide health professionals with up to date information on nutrition and nutrition-related disorders in order to enable them to continuously improve patient care based on the latest medical and scientific breakthroughs.

One of the key pillars of the Nestlé Nutrition Institute is the *Annales Nestlé*, a pediatric journal that has been published on a regular basis since 1942. It contains review articles on clinical practice and research in all fields of pediatrics with focus on nutrition. Each publication deals with one specific topic, such as diabetes mellitus, HIV and nutrition or infant growth. The *Annales Nestlé* comprises 3 issues each year in 3 languages (English, French and Spanish), and with around 50,000 copies per issue is one of the most widely read pediatric journals in the world.

The *Annales Nestlé* is edited by an independent editorial board of six highly respected professors of pediatrics, thus guaranteeing the medical and scientific impartiality of the journal, and hence the high level of respect and appreciation in medical and scientific circles. The editorial board sets editorial policy, identifies topics to be addressed, selects authors and assesses the articles' contents.

The *Annales Nestlé* are published by S. Karger AG, one of the world's most highly respected scientific and medical publishers.

Prof. Ferdinand Haschke, MD, PhD
Chairman
Nestlé Nutrition Institute
Vevey (Switzerland)

KARGER

Fax +41 61 306 12 34
E-Mail karger@karger.ch
www.karger.com

Access to full text and tables of contents, including tentative ones for forthcoming issues: www.karger.com/ane_issues

Annales Nestlé

Ann Nestlé [Engl] 2010;68:5–6
DOI: 10.1159/000298778

Editorial

Eating for Two?

Yes, pregnant women are eating for two, but the equation is not as simple as the statement suggests. Hormonal changes in the mother drive a number of metabolic and physiological processes that are designed to support the development and growth of the fetus, without undue burden on the mother. As a result the increased nutrient requirements of pregnancy are not simply the sum of those accumulated by the fetus, the placenta and by maternal tissues. Rather, hormonal changes are designed to increase the delivery of nutrition to the fetus such that the actual energy requirement during the first trimester of pregnancy is not increased from the nonpregnant state and maternal energy intake in the second and third trimesters only requires an increase in energy intake by about 10%. However, in cases where the nutritional fuel is insufficient or in excess, metabolic and physiological adaptations result and these adaptations often have long-lasting consequences.

A relevant and contemporary example in which the depletion of a specific nutrient during early pregnancy causes permanent long-term consequences is that of folate and neural tube defects (NTDs). NTDs are congenital malformations which arise during the development of the brain and spinal cord. A band of cells along the dorsal surface of the embryo develops into a groove and then a hollow tube. The process is completed within a month of fertilization (by the 6th week after the last menstrual period). Incomplete closure of the neural tube causes NTDs. Exactly why NTDs happen is not entirely clear, although both environmental and genetic factors are considered important, including the role of folate in ameliorating the effects of disturbed homocysteine metabolism. The Cochrane systematic review on the topic [1] has summarized the results of 4 trials involving 6,425 women and showed that preconception folate supplementation reduced the incidence of NTDs by 72% (relative risk = 0.28, 95% confidence interval = 0.13–0.58), clearly highlighting the strong protective effect of folate supplementation and the rationale of the public health recommendation for universal periconceptional supplementation for all women.

This issue of *Annales Nestlé* is dedicated to mother-child nutrition and has a particular focus on pregnancy nutrition with 3 papers that highlight the importance of balanced nutrition in both industrialized and semi-industrialized environments.

The first, by Professor Cetin and Dr Cardellicchio from the Mother and Child Hospital Luigi Sacco and University of Milan, provides an instructive overview of metabolic interplay between the mother, the placenta and the fetus, and how changes in the equilibrium between mother, placenta and fetus can compromise the pregnancy outcome. Clearly maternal diet is an important environmental factor, but it is not the only one. Maternal body composition, maternal hormonal adaptations, the quality and function of the placenta and even the fetus through its unique genetic makeup and endocrine environment all contribute to the quality of the pregnancy outcome.

The second chapter by Dr Herring, Temple University Philadelphia, and Dr Oken, Harvard Medical School, strongly complements the first with a detailed review of

KARGER

Fax +41 61 306 12 34
E-Mail karger@karger.ch
www.karger.com

0517–8606/10/0681–0005$26.00/0

Accessible online at:
www.karger.com/ane

the influences of gestational weight gain on both maternal and child outcomes. The chapter summarizes the clinical and epidemiological evidence linking gestational weight gain with glucose metabolism, hypertensive disorders, complications at birth, postpartum weight retention, maternal obesity risk and the associated cardiometabolic sequelae, as well as fetal growth, preterm birth and infant mortality, and longer-term weight and obesity risk in the offspring. The chapter has important messages for both industrialized and semi-industrialized countries as both low and high gestational weight gains are associated with negative outcomes. Herring and Oken end with an excellent state-of-the-art summary of the gestational weight gain targets for women entering pregnancy with low, normal and high body mass indices.

The final chapter by Dr Usha Ramakrishnan from Emory University, Atlanta, provides a critical review of the effectiveness of prenatal nutrient supplements in improving maternal and child health outcomes. The range of supplements reviewed includes iron and folic acid, multiple micronutrients, calcium, magnesium, iodine, vitamin A, zinc, vitamin D, antioxidants, ω–3 long-chain polyunsaturated fatty acids and probiotics. The theme regarding the different needs of women from industrialized and semi-industrialized communities recurs. This time the benefit of multiple micronutrient supplements and minerals such as calcium and zinc during pregnancy for at-risk populations is shown to promote the health and well-being of mothers and their offspring in a cost-effective manner.

This issue of *Annales Nestlé* has not dealt with nutrition during lactation, where the delivery of nutrients is optimized through breast milk; this could be a topic for a later issue.

Olle Hernell, Umeå
Michael Lentze, Bonn
Maria Makrides, Adelaide
Frank Ruemmele, Paris
Noel Solomons, Guatemala City
Hania Szajewska, Warsaw

Reference

1 Lumley J, Watson L, Watson M, Bower C: Periconceptional supplementation with folate and/or multivitamins for preventing neural tube defects. Cochrane Database Syst Rev 2001;3:CD001056.

Annales Nestlé

Ann Nestlé [Engl] 2010;68:7–15
DOI: 10.1159/000298779

Physiology of Pregnancy: Interaction between Mother and Child

Overview of the Nutritional Interaction between the Mother and Fetus

Irene Cetin   Manuela Cardellicchio

Department of Mother and Child, Hospital Luigi Sacco, and Centre for Fetal Research Giorgio Pardi, University of Milan, Milan, Italy

Key Words
Fetal growth · Fetal nutrition · Pregnancy · Metabolism · Placenta transport

Abstract
In the last years evidence has shown how lifelong well-being strongly depends on intrauterine growth and development during intrauterine life. Fetal growth can achieve its full potential only with an adequate and fine-tuned interaction between mother, placenta and fetus. Several environmental and maternal factors like maternal diet, body composition and endocrine status may alter this delicate equilibrium. Moreover, placental function and metabolism contribute and regulate the availability of fetal nutrients. Changes in this complex mechanism may compromise the pregnancy outcome. In this chapter we wish to elucidate the physiologic mechanisms that regulate this interaction and how also little modifications may predispose to pathologies like intrauterine growth restriction and gestational diabetes with important consequences on fetal and adult health.

Introduction

Not too long ago, pregnancy was considered a 9-month period during which the mothers were free to eat 'for two' in order to have a healthy and strong baby. In recent years, after countless studies, this point of view has changed and it has become clearer that beyond a balanced maternal diet, other factors strongly influence fetal development. Pregnancy can actually be considered as a 3-compartment model where mother, placenta and fetus interact to guarantee fetal growth and development (fig. 1).

This chapter aims to elucidate the mechanisms at the basis of this interaction and how perturbations of this equilibrium may compromise the pregnancy outcome.

The Mother

Together with genes, the main determinant of fetal growth is the availability of nutrients reaching the fetus through the umbilical vein. These nutrients are transferred from the mother through the placenta but the nutrient composition in maternal blood is dependent on

KARGER

Fax +41 61 306 12 34
E-Mail karger@karger.ch
www.karger.com

0517–8606/10/0681–0007$26.00/0

Accessible online at:
www.karger.com/ane

Irene Cetin
Department of Mother and Child, Hospital Luigi Sacco, University of Milan
Via G. B. Grassi 74
IT–20157 Milan (Italy)
Tel. +39 02 3904 2264, E-Mail irene.cetin@unimi.it

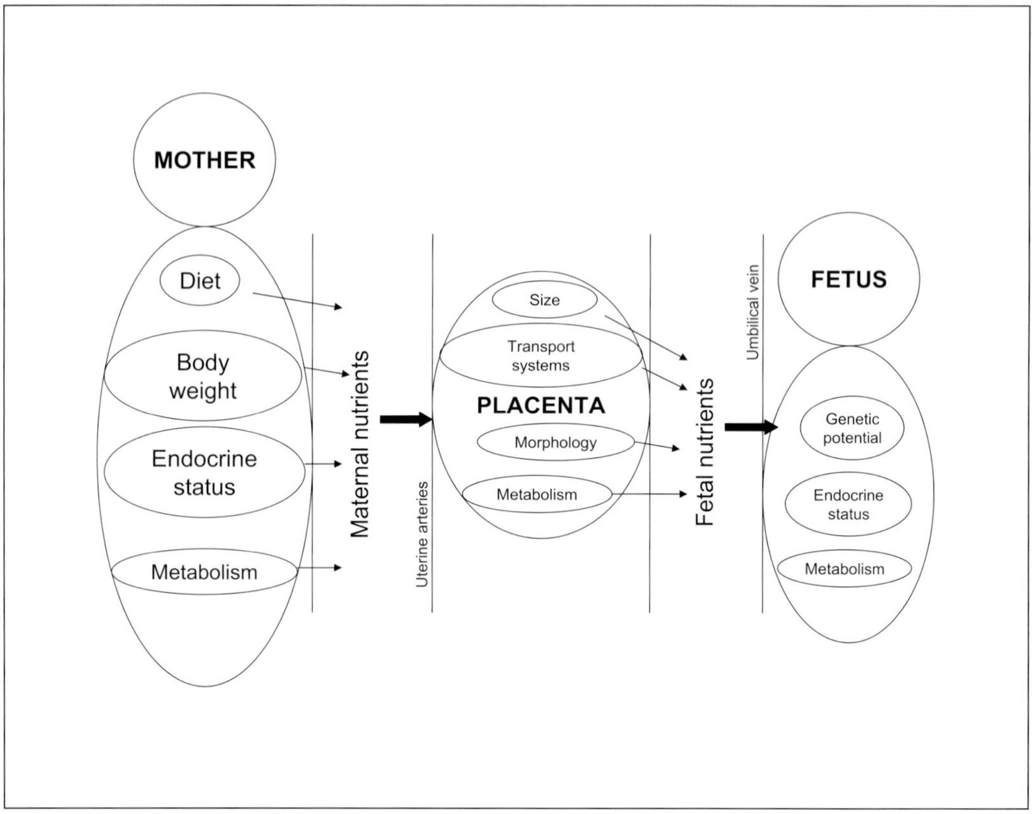

Fig. 1. Pregnancy: 3-compartment model.

various maternal factors: diet, body composition, endocrine status and metabolism.

Maternal Diet

Diet is recognized as one of the major environmental factors influencing the development of the embryo and the fetus as well as maternal health. Each stage in embryonic and fetal development is influenced by maternal nutrients and the timing of a nutritional insult impacts differently on the nature of adult diseases by programming the postnatal pathophysiology, thus indicating that the early environment modifies the expression of the genome. On the whole, early programming is an established concept in biology: prenatal sex hormone exposure determines gender development (i.e. endocrine programming), perinatal exposure to allergens may induce tolerance (i.e. immunological programming), and monoallelic expression regulated by differential DNA methylation induces Prader-Willi syndrome, Angelman syndrome and others (i.e. epigenetic programming).

Therefore, programming of human adult functions and diseases seems to be influenced by hormones, metabolites and neurotransmitters during critical developmental periods as well as the early nutrition [1]. In fact, undernutrition of animals at early but not at later ages determines adult body size [2], and the developmental origins of adult disease seem to be related to poor fetal nutrition and low birth weight [3]. Evidence of the relationship between nutrition in early life and lifelong health exists for cardiovascular risk, infection and allergy risk, autoimmune diseases (e.g. diabetes type 1, inflammatory bowel disease, celiac disease), bone health, neural and brain function, as well as obesity.

Pregnancy leads to a modest increase in energy requirements compared to the nonpregnant status: 375, 1,200 and 1,950 kJ/day in the first, second and third trimester, respectively [4]. These additional calories can be met by a modest increase in consumption of a balanced diet (20–35% of fats, 15–20% of proteins, 40–50% of carbohydrates). A balanced maternal diet is fundamental

Table 1. Animal and human studies about nutrient impact on pregnancy outcome

Elevated glucose levels in diabetic mothers	Altered blastocyst development and implantation	Leunda-Casi et al. [74], 2001, [75], 2002
High dietary intake of saturated fatty acid	Elevated risk of fetal outflow tract defects	Smedts et al. [76], 2008
	Elevated risk of cardiovascular disease in adult life	Chechi et al. [7], 2006, [8], 2009
High intake of western diet	Elevated risk of lip and palate cleft	Vujkovic et al. [77], 2007
Depletion of maternal folate intake	Elevated risk of IUGR	Van Eijsden et al. [78], 2008
	Elevated risk of preterm delivery and fetal malformations	Czeizel et al. [79], 1999 Tamura and Picciano [80], 2006
Inadequate maternal iron intake	Elevated risk of preterm delivery	Zhou et al. [81], 1998
Reduced maternal dietary intake of B vitamins	Elevated risk of congenital heart defects	Verkleij-Hagoort et al. [82], 2006

not only to fetal development during pregnancy but also to the offspring's long-term health.

In recent years, it has become clear that maternal diet is relevant not only during pregnancy but already before conception. In particular, the periconceptional period is a critical step in determining fetal development and health. The onset of several malformations and pregnancy-related disorders (i.e., congenital abnormalities, fetal loss, miscarriage, insufficient fetal growth, premature birth, preeclampsia) may indeed occur during this period, in particular when micronutrient imbalances occur [5, 6] (table 1).

While in developed countries pregnant women can choose any kind of food based on their personal taste, in poor countries women may be exposed to undernutrition, but in both cases, an unbalanced diet may have dramatic consequences. Animal studies have shown that an excessive consumption of saturated fatty acids during pregnancy may permanently alter the fetal lipid metabolism in adult life, increasing the risk for cardiovascular disease [7, 8]. Recently, Howie et al. [9] reported that offspring born by rat dams fed with a high-fat diet are smaller and are predisposed to developing obesity independently of postnatal diet.

The Dutch famine that occurred during the Second World War allowed the study of maternal undernutrition showing that when severe maternal undernutrition occurs in the second and third trimester, it affects the birth weight, whereas compensatory placental growth was able to maintain a normal birth weight when undernutrition occurred in the first trimester [10]. Similarly to what occurs with overnutrition, individuals exposed to undernutrition in utero have an increased prevalence of cardiovascular disease [11], diabetes [12, 13] and obesity [14].

Therefore, it is fundamental that women of reproductive age and pregnant women are counseled to consume wholesome foods as well as a diversified range of foods in the right quantities, to avoid under- and overnutrition as well as micronutrient imbalances.

Body Composition

Pregravidic weight is an important factor influencing the fetal and pregnancy outcome. In particular, the maternal body mass index (BMI) is one of the best markers of nutritional status. The World Health Organization guidelines define overweight as BMI 25–29.9, obesity as BMI $\geq$30 and underweight as BMI <19.8.

Today, obesity is a major burden in developed countries. Its incidence ranges from 18.5 to 38.3% among pregnant women in the USA [15]. Maternal obesity is associated with increased maternal and neonatal risks for pregnancy diseases such as preeclampsia, gestational diabetes, caesarean section, low Apgar scores, macrosomia and neural tube defects [15, 16]. Obese women have higher blood concentrations of nutrients due to lower insulin sensitivity [17]; increased substrates are then available for placental transfer to the fetus and contribute to fetal overgrowth (fig. 2).

On the other hand, maternal underweight is associated with increased risks of preterm labor, intrauterine growth restriction (IUGR), low birth weight and maternal anemia, this last probably due to deficiencies of micronutrients like iron and folic acid [18, 19].

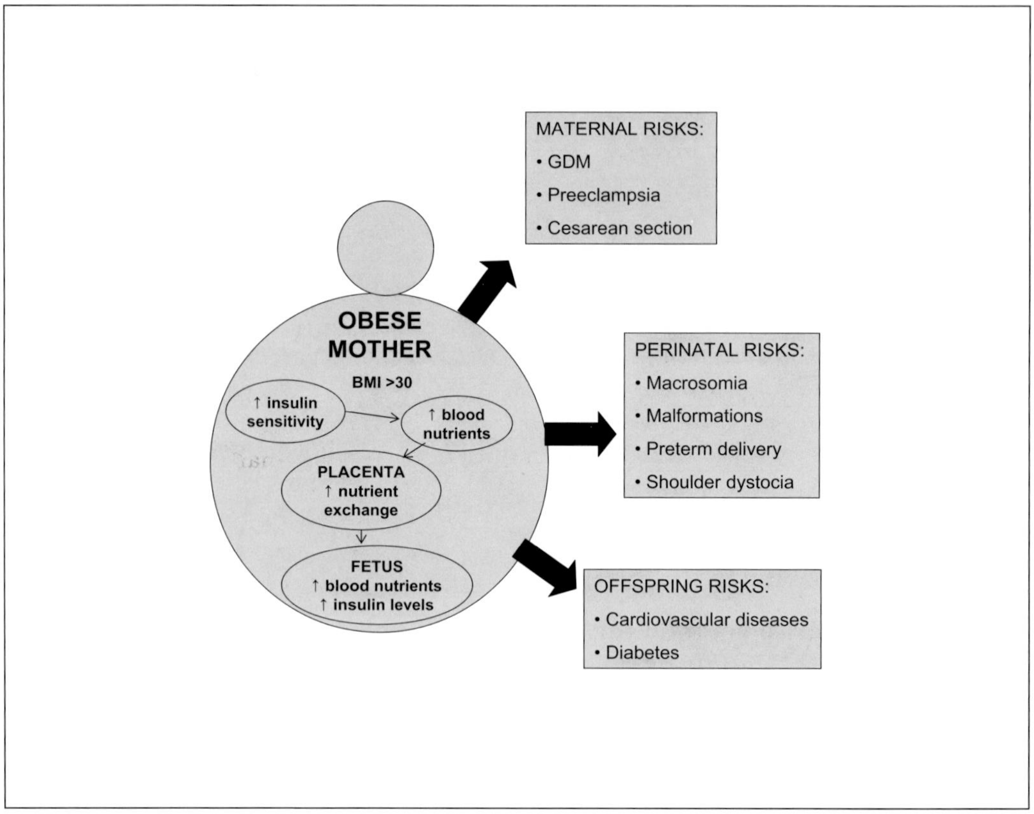

Fig. 2. Effects of obesity on pregnancy, fetus and offspring.

Therefore, both underweight and obese mothers are at increased risk of adverse perinatal outcome. Major efforts should be made to reduce these risks by encouraging a nutritional education program for women of childbearing age and for pregnant women of different social and educational levels.

Endocrinology and Metabolism

From the beginning of pregnancy, maternal metabolism undergoes a number of changes to adapt to fetal and placental needs. In the first trimester these needs are mainly qualitative for organ development, since embryonic growth is still limited. In this period, hyperphagia and rise in insulin sensitivity allow the mother to store fats in the adipose tissue and to increase her net body weight [20]. This anabolic status occurs even in conditions of malnutrition [21, 22].

In the third trimester fetal growth becomes exponential and at the same time fetal nutritional demands increase. In order to adapt to this new condition, the maternal metabolism switches to a catabolic status: progesterone, cortisol, prolactin and leptin lead to a decrease in insulin responsiveness [23, 24] with a consequent increase in free fatty acids and glycerol plasma levels. Increased concentrations of maternal substrates are now available to cross the placenta and reach the fetus.

This physiologic adaptation is enhanced in pregnancies complicated by gestational diabetes where insulin sensitivity is significantly reduced, leading to higher maternal concentrations of glucose and free fatty acids. Obesity is an independent risk factor for developing gestational diabetes mellitus (GDM). Obese mothers have a 3 times higher risk of developing GDM compared to non-obese mothers [25, 26]. Today, the prevalence of obesity and consequently of GDM is rising worldwide together with maternal and fetal complications [25]. GDM as well as obesity predispose both mother and child to develop the metabolic syndrome and to a higher risk of cardiovascular disease [27].

The Placenta

Placental function is one of the major factors able to determine fetal nutrition and growth. This organ is not an inert membrane, since it regulates nutrients and oxygen flow to the fetus both quantitatively and qualitatively through its transport systems and its metabolism [20, 28]. The role of the placenta is shown in pathologic conditions of altered fetal growth like IUGR and GDM, both characterized by specific placenta phenotypes [29].

Implantation and placentation begin in the first days of pregnancy and continue throughout gestation. During this long period, the structure and function of the placenta undergo important changes to meet fetal demands: progressive increases in surface area, decreases in thickness [30, 20] and modification of nutrient transport systems.

The transfer capacity of the placenta is dependent on its size, morphology, blood flow and abundance of transporters [31]. Moreover, the placenta also influences the rate of fetal growth with its capacity to synthesize hormones and metabolize nutrients [32].

Size, Morphology and Metabolism

At midpregnancy, the placenta uses half of the oxygen and glucose received from maternal circulation for its own growth and metabolism, whereas in the second half of pregnancy it transfers the majority of nutrients to the fetus [33]. Its efficiency is defined as grams of fetus produced per gram of placenta [34] and in human beings this value is approximately 5:1 near term gestation [35]. The fetal/placental weight ratio is genetically determined, but it can be modified by environmental conditions during pregnancy [36]. Experimental animal studies have demonstrated that placental efficiency is reduced by decreases in uterine blood flow or by hypoxemia, while dietary calorie or protein deprivation leads to an increased efficiency in the first part of gestation and to a decreased efficiency closer to term [37, 38]. Generally, in normal oxygenation conditions lighter placentae are more efficient than heavier ones in humans [36].

In early stages of placental development branches of uterine arteries are converted into low-resistance vessels by placental extravillous trophoblast [39]. IUGR pregnancy is characterized by an incomplete spiral artery invasion and consequently by a condition of hypoxia and hypoperfusion. However, placentae of IUGR are characterized by a decreased coefficient of oxygen extraction and by increased uterine venous O_2 content, suggesting an inability of fetal villi to extract oxygen independently of blood flow [40]. Actually, IUGR placentae are characterized by an abnormal pattern of villous morphology and by increased thickness of the exchange barrier and both of these abnormalities seem to reduce oxygen and nutrient permeability [29]. Recent data show that the mitochondrial DNA content is significantly increased in IUGR placentae and that this increase is inversely related to umbilical venous oxygen [41]. Increased placental mitochondrial DNA may either represent a compensatory mechanism to hypoxia or a placental metabolic adaptation to the reduced nutrient availability.

An increased placental/fetal weight ratio has been reported in pregnancies complicated by GDM even with an optimal maternal glycemic control [42]. The increased placental mass could augment nutrient exchange by extending the surface area available for substrate transfer.

Transport Systems

Glucose, the most important and essential nutrient for fetal growth, is transported from mother to fetus by a facilitated diffusion system and its fetal concentration is constantly lower and dependent on maternal concentration and gestational age [43].

Amino acids are transported by active carriers, in particular neutral amino acids, by a sodium-dependent transport system, while branched amino acids, phenylalanine and lysine are carried by a sodium-independent transporter [44]. During pregnancy, the fetal amino acid concentrations are constantly higher than in the mother [45]. Stable isotope studies have shown that fetal nonessential amino acids (i.e. glycine and proline) mainly derive from placental production from metabolically related amino acids. In particular, for glycine and serine and for glutamate and glutamine an interorgan cycle between placenta and fetal liver has been hypothesized [46, 47], while maternal essential amino acids are taken up by the placenta and reach the fetus quite rapidly in bolus studies [46, 47].

Recently Jansson et al. [48] have suggested that the placenta is a 'nutrient sensor' able to modify its transport function according to maternal nutrient supply and fetal needs.

Fatty acids can cross the placenta as free fatty acids by simple diffusion or as lipoproteins connecting specific binding proteins and are then released by way of specific placenta lipoprotein lipases [49]. Simple diffusion is allowed by the presence of a maternal-fetal concentration gradient. The fetal concentration is constantly lower than in the mother but also qualitatively different: long-chain polyunsaturated fatty acids (LCPUFA) like arachidonic

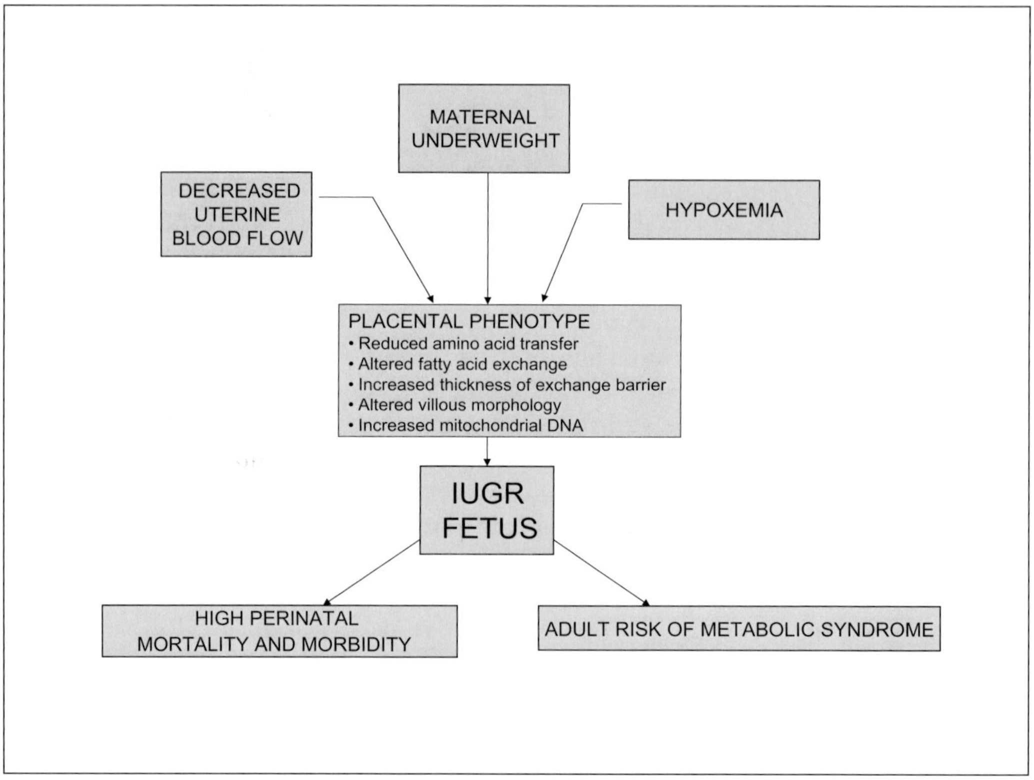

Fig. 3. Pathophysiology of IUGR.

acid and docosahexaenoic acid are present in higher proportions compared to their precursors linoleic acid and α-linolenic acid [50]. This phenomenon, called 'biomagnification', is due to the ability of the placenta to transfer preferentially LCPUFA to guarantee a correct fetal neurodevelopment, but the underlying mechanism is still not clear [51].

IUGR, a condition characterized by the inability of the fetus to achieve its full growth potential [28], is an important cause of perinatal mortality and morbidity, and it increases the risk of developing cardiovascular diseases in adult life (fig. 3) [52]. Placental metabolism and nutrient transport systems are altered in IUGR placentae [29]: the fetal amino acid concentrations are reduced in IUGR fetuses [53] and a reduction in the activity of a number of amino acid transport systems has been demonstrated by some studies [54]. The total plasma levels of fatty acids are the same in IUGR fetuses [55], but the relative composition is different, with a significantly lower fetal/maternal ratio for the LCPUFA docosahexaenoic acid and arachidonic acid [56]. These changes may explain the high susceptibility of IUGR fetuses to vascular brain damage.

GDM pregnancies are characterized by fetal overgrowth due to an increase in nutrient availability. However, in the last years, it has been shown that the risk of excessive fetal growth is elevated also with a strict maternal metabolic control [57]. This evidence, together with in vitro studies, suggests that even short periods of metabolic imbalance early in pregnancy may affect placenta transport systems [58]. Neutral amino acid transporters are markedly increased in the syncytiotrophoblast of GDM pregnancies, whereas the glucose transport system is upregulated only in pregnancies complicated by diabetes mellitus type 1 but not in GDM [59, 60].

Data obtained in GDM pregnancies at the time of cesarean section show that the fetal glucose levels are higher than in normal pregnancies even when the mother has glucose levels in the normal range. In these same pregnancies, the fetal oxygen levels are decreased and the lactate concentrations increased, confirming placental alterations [61]. Moreover, the fetal concentrations of most amino acids are significantly increased in GDM pregnancies [62].

Table 2. Imprinted genes involved in fetal growth

Gnas	Chromosome 2	Cattanach et al. [83], 2000
Peg 1	Chromosome 6	Coan et al. [84], 2005
Peg 3	Chromosome 7	
Peg 10	Chromosome 6	
Grb 10	Chromosome 11	
Gtl 2	Chromosome 12	
Rtl 1	Chromosome 12	
Igf 2	Chromosome 7	Bressan et al. [85], 2009
Slc238a4	Chromosome 15	
Dlk 1	Chromosome 12	
Plagl 1	Chromosome 10	

The marked insulin resistance of GDM and the consequently enhanced lipolysis determines a high-fat maternal-fetal concentration gradient and then a higher transfer of fatty acids to the fetus. This transfer is favored also by an increased expression of a specific fatty-acid-binding protein (L-FABP) on microvillus membrane [63].

The Fetus

The fetus receives a nutrient mix that is determined by the mother and the placenta. Both are able to influence the fetal diet and consequently fetal daily growth. However, the fetus is also a key player in its own development through its genes and the endocrine environment. Besides traditional mendelian genetic inheritance, some inherited genes, called imprinted genes, act differently in relation to their maternal or paternal belonging (table 2). Maternal genes act as growth suppressors, whereas paternal ones are growth promoters, so an imbalance in their expression may alter fetal and placental growth, as shown in uniparental disomy [64].

Different environmental conditions, like maternal diet or uterine blood flow, influence fetal growth and can compromise this genetic potential. The fetus's endocrine status is changed and the placental efficiency influenced by these insults. In particular under favorable conditions, the fetus enhances anabolic hormones like insulin and insulin-like growth factors (IGFs), whereas under adverse conditions catabolic hormones like cortisol and cathecolamines increase [32].

Among the hormones, IGFs seems to have a predominant role in regulating fetal growth: they are expressed from both maternal and fetal tissues and are able to regulate placental efficiency by modifying its transfer ability. Animal and in vitro studies show that placental weight, thickness and surface area are directly related to maternal IGF-I concentrations [65, 66]. In the human placenta, maternal IGF-1 increases the amino acid uptake [67]. Fetal IGF-I instead seems to be involved in fetal but not in placental growth: mice with deletion of the *Igf-I* gene develop growth restriction [68].

Igf-II is also implicated in fetoplacental development: its overexpression determines fetal and placental overgrowth, whereas its deletion provokes growth restriction [69]. IGF-II production is regulated by an imprinted gene with paternal expression. In Igf-II KO mice both fetal and placental weights are strongly reduced with significant changes in placental amino acid transport systems happening already at midpregnancy [70]. The real molecular mechanisms at the basis of the ability of IGFs to influence fetal and placental growth are still not clear, but recent data suggest that they may regulate placental transporter concentrations by influencing the mTOR pathway [71].

Moreover, when the fetal nutrient exchange is altered, the fetus may also modify its own metabolism in order to try to adapt to the adverse environment. In particular, preliminary data in IUGR fetuses indicate a significantly lower umbilical oxygen uptake value on per kilogram basis, suggesting that their metabolic rate is significantly decreased [72].

On the other side of the fetal growth spectrum, fetuses of GDM mothers show reduced levels of arachidonic (20:4 n–6) and docosahexaenoic (22:6 n–3) acids. Recent data show that this difference is evident in the umbilical artery but not in the umbilical vein, therefore suggesting changes in fetal metabolism of LCPUFA rather than altered placental transfer [73].

Conclusions

When external factors hinder the fetal genetic growth potential, both fetus and placenta start morphological and functional adaptation mechanisms to reduce the imbalance. However, when these compensatory changes are insufficient, growth restriction or overgrowth are established with consequent intrauterine and adult health disorders.

References

1 Lucas A: Programming by early nutrition in man. Ciba Found Symp 1991;156:38–50; discussion 50–55.
2 Widdowson EM, McCance RA: Use of random specimens of urine to compare dietary intakes of African and British children. Arch Dis Child 1970;45:547–552.
3 Hales CN, Barker DJ: Type 2 (non-insulin-dependent) diabetes mellitus: the thrifty phenotype hypothesis. Diabetologia 1992; 35:595–601.
4 Butte NF, King JC: Energy requirements during pregnancy and lactation (review). Public Health Nutr 2005;8:1010–1027.
5 Steegers EAP: Begin at the beginning: some reflections on future periconceptional and obstetric care and research in the Netherlands. Eur Clin Obstet Gynaecol 2005;1:203–214, DOI 10.1007/s11296-005-0011-8.
6 Cetin I, Berti C, Calabrese S: Role of micronutrients in the periconceptional period. Hum Reprod Update 2010;16:80–95.
7 Chechi K, Cheema SK: Maternal diet rich in saturated fats has deleterious effects on plasma lipids of mice. Exp Clin Cardiol 2006;11: 129–135.
8 Chechi K, McGuire JJ, Cheema SK: Developmental programming of lipid metabolism and aortic vascular function in C57BL/6 mice: a novel study suggesting an involvement of LDL-receptor. Am J Physiol Regul Integr Comp Physiol 2009;296:R1029–R1040.
9 Howie GJ, Sloboda DM, Kamal T, Vickers MH: Maternal nutritional history predicts obesity in adult offspring independent of postnatal diet. J Physiol 2009;587:905–915.
10 Stein Z, Susser M: The Dutch famine, 1944–1945, and the reproductive process. I. Effects or six indices at birth. Pediatr Res 1975;9:70–76.
11 Painter RC, de Rooij SR, Bossuyt PM, Simmers TA, Osmond C, Barker DJ, Bleker OP, Roseboom TJ: Early onset of coronary artery disease after prenatal exposure to the Dutch famine. Am J Clin Nutr 2006;84:322–327; quiz 466–467.
12 De Rooij SR, Painter RC, Roseboom TJ, Phillips DI, Osmond C, Barker DJ, Tanck MW, Michels RP, Bossuyt PM, Bleker OP: Glucose tolerance at age 58 and the decline of glucose tolerance in comparison with age 50 in people prenatally exposed to the Dutch famine. Diabetologia 2006;49:637–643.
13 Ravelli AC, van der Meulen JH, Michels RP, Osmond C, Barker DJ, Hales CN, Bleker OP: Glucose tolerance in adults after prenatal exposure to famine. Lancet 1998;351:173–177.
14 Ravelli AC, van der Meulen JH, Osmond C, Barker DJ, Bleker OP: Obesity at the age of 50 years in men and women exposed to famine prenatally. Am J Clin Nutr 1999;70:811–816.
15 Galtier-Dereure F, Boegner C, Bringer J: Obesity and pregnancy: complications and cost (review). Am J Clin Nutr 2000;71(suppl 5):1242S–1248S.
16 Doherty DA, Magann EF, Francis J, Morrison JC, Newnham JP: Pre-pregnancy body mass index and pregnancy outcomes. Int J Gynaecol Obstet 2006;95:242–247.
17 King JC: Maternal obesity, metabolism, and pregnancy outcomes (review). Annu Rev Nutr 2006;26:271–291.
18 Ehrenberg HM, Huston-Presley L, Catalano PM: The influence of obesity and gestational diabetes mellitus on accretion and the distribution of adipose tissue in pregnancy. Am J Obstet Gynecol 2003;189:944–948.
19 Sahu MT, Agarwal A, Das V, Pandey A: Impact of maternal body mass index on obstetric outcome. J Obstet Gynaecol Res 2007;33: 655–659.
20 Cetin I, Alvino G, Radaelli T, Pardi G: Fetal nutrition: a review. Acta Paediatr Suppl 2005;94:7–13.
21 Prentice AM, Goldberg GR: Energy adaptations in human pregnancy: limits and long-term consequences (review). Am J Clin Nutr 2000;71(suppl 5):1226S–1232S.
22 Herrera E: Lipid metabolism in pregnancy and its consequences in the fetus and newborn (review). Endocrine 2002;19:43–55.
23 Catov JM, Patrick TE, Powers RW, Ness RB, Harger G, Roberts JM: Maternal leptin across pregnancy in women with small-for-gestational-age infants. Am J Obstet Gynecol 2007;196:558.e1–e8.
24 Cousins L: Insulin sensitivity in pregnancy. Diabetes 1991;40:39–43.
25 Yogev Y, Catalano PM: Pregnancy and obesity (review). Obstet Gynecol Clin North Am 2009;36:285–300, viii.
26 Bianco AT, Smilen SW, Davis Y, Lopez S, Lapinski R, Lockwood CJ: Pregnancy outcome and weight gain recommendations for the morbidly obese woman. Obstet Gynecol 1998;91:97–102.
27 Verma A, Boney CM, Tucker R, Vohr BR: Insulin resistance syndrome in women with prior history of gestational diabetes mellitus. J Clin Endocrinol Metab 2002;87:3227–3235.
28 Cetin I, Alvino G: Intrauterine growth restriction: implications for placental metabolism and transport – a review. Placenta 2009; 30(suppl A):S77–S82.
29 Sibley CP, Turner MA, Cetin I, Ayuk P, Boyd CA, D'Souza SW, Glazier JD, Greenwood SL, Jansson T, Powell T: Placental phenotypes of intrauterine growth. Pediatr Res 2005;58: 827–832.
30 Kaufmann P, Sheffer I: Placental development; in Polin RA, Fox WW (eds): Fetal and Neonatal Physiology, ed 2. Philadelphia, Saunders, 1998, pp 59–70.
31 Fowden AL, Sibley C, Reik W, Constancia M: Imprinted genes, placental development and fetal growth (review). Horm Res 2006; 65(suppl 3):50–58.
32 Fowden AL, Forhead AJ: Endocrine mechanisms of intrauterine programming (review). Reproduction 2004;127:515–526.
33 Bell AW, Kennaugh JM, Battaglia FC, Makowski EL, Meschia G: Metabolic and circulatory studies of fetal lamb at midgestation. Am J Physiol 1986;250:E538–E544.
34 Wilson ME, Ford SP: Comparative aspects of placental efficiency (review). Reprod Suppl 2001;58:223–232.
35 Leiser R, Kaufmann P: Placental structure: in a comparative aspect. Exp Clin Endocrinol 1994;102:122–134.
36 Fowden AL, Sferruzzi-Perri AN, Coan PM, Constancia M, Burton GJ: Placental efficiency and adaptation: endocrine regulation (review). J Physiol 2009;587:3459–3472.
37 Woodall SM, Johnston BM, Breier BH, Gluckman PD: Chronic maternal undernutrition in the rat leads to delayed postnatal growth and elevated blood pressure of offspring. Pediatr Res 1996;40:438–443.
38 Vaughn PR, Lobo C, Battaglia FC, Fennessey PV, Wilkening RB, Meschia G: Glutamine-glutamate exchange between placenta and fetal liver. Am J Physiol 1995;268:E705–E711.
39 Huppertz B, Peeters LL: Vascular biology in implantation and placentation (review). Angiogenesis 2005;8:157–167.
40 Pardi G, Cetin I, Marconi AM, Lanfranchi A, Bozzetti P, Ferrazzi E, Buscaglia M, Battaglia FC: Diagnostic value of blood sampling in fetuses with growth retardation. N Engl J Med 1993;328:692–696.
41 Lattuada D, Colleoni F, Martinelli A, Garretto A, Magni R, Radaelli T, Cetin I: Higher mitochondrial DNA content in human IUGR placenta. Placenta 2008;29:1029–1033.
42 Taricco E, Radaelli T, Nobile de Santis MS, Cetin I: Foetal and placental weights in relation to maternal characteristics in gestational diabetes. Placenta 2003;24:343–347.
43 Marconi AM, Paolini C, Buscaglia M, Zerbe G, Battaglia FC, Pardi G: The impact of gestational age and fetal growth on the maternal-fetal glucose concentration difference. Obstet Gynecol 1996;87:937–942.
44 Cetin I, de Santis MS, Taricco E, Radaelli T, Teng C, Ronzoni S, Spada E, Milani S, Pardi G: Maternal and fetal amino acid concentrations in normal pregnancies and in pregnancies with gestational diabetes mellitus. Am J Obstet Gynecol 2005;192:610–617.
45 Cetin I, Ronzoni S, Marconi AM, Perugino G, Corbetta C, Battaglia FC, Pardi G: Maternal concentrations and fetal-maternal concentration differences of plasma amino acids in normal and intrauterine growth-restricted pregnancies. Am J Obstet Gynecol 1996; 174:1575–1583.

46 Cetin I, Marconi AM, Baggiani AM, Buscaglia M, Pardi G, Fennessey PV, Battaglia FC: In vivo placental transport of glycine and leucine in human pregnancies. Pediatr Res 1995;37:571–575.
47 Paolini CL, Marconi AM, Ronzoni S, Di Noio M, Fennessey PV, Pardi G, Battaglia FC: Placental transport of leucine, phenylalanine, glycine, and proline in intrauterine growth-restricted pregnancies. J Clin Endocrinol Metab 2001;86:5427–5432.
48 Jansson T, Powell TL: IFPA 2005 Award in Placentology Lecture. Human placental transport in altered fetal growth: does the placenta function as a nutrient sensor? A review. Placenta 2006;27(suppl A):S91–S97.
49 Herrera E, Amusquivar E, Lopez-Soldado I, Ortega H: Maternal lipid metabolism and placental lipid transfer. Horm Res 2006; 65(suppl 3):59–64.
50 Crawford MA, Hassan AG, Williams G & Whitehouse WL: Essential fatty acids and fetal brain growth. Lancet 1976;1:452–453.
51 Cetin I, Koletzko B: Long-chain ω-3 fatty acid supply in pregnancy and lactation (review). Curr Opin Clin Nutr Metab Care 2008;11:297–302.
52 Murphy VE, Smith R, Giles WB, Clifton VL: Endocrine regulation of human fetal growth: the role of the mother, placenta, and fetus (review). Endocr Rev 2006;27:141–169.
53 Cetin I, Corbetta C, Sereni LP, Marconi AM, Bozzetti P, Pardi G, Battaglia FC: Umbilical amino acid concentrations in normal and growth-retarded fetuses sampled in utero by cordocentesis Am J Obstet Gynecol 1990; 162:253–261.
54 Jansson T, Ekstrand Y, Björn C, Wennergren M, Powell TL: Alterations in the activity of placental amino acid transporters in pregnancies complicated by diabetes. Diabetes 2002;51:2214–2219.
55 Cetin I, Giovannini N, Alvino G, Agostoni C, Riva E, Giovannini M, Pardi G: Intrauterine growth restriction is associated with changes in polyunsaturated fatty acid fetal-maternal relationships. Pediatr Res 2002;52: 750–755.
56 Cetin I, Alvino G, Cardellicchio M: Long-chain polyunsaturated fatty acids and dietary fats in fetal nutrition J Physiol 2009; 587:3441–3451.
57 Ericsson A, Saljo K, Sjostrand E, Jansson N, Prasad PD, Powell TL, Jansson T: Brief hyperglycaemia in the early pregnant rat increases fetal weight at term by stimulating placental growth and affecting placental nutrient transport. J Physiol 2007;581:1323–1332.
58 Jansson T, Cetin I, Powell TL, Desoye G, Radaelli T, Ericsson A, Sibley CP: Placental transport and metabolism in fetal overgrowth – a workshop report. Placenta 2006; 27(suppl A):S109–S113.
59 Jansson T: Amino acid transporters in the human placenta (review) . Pediatr Res 2001; 49:141–147.
60 Jansson T, Ylvén K, Wennergren M, Powell TL: Glucose transport and system A activity in syncytiotrophoblast microvillous and basal plasma membranes in intrauterine growth restriction. Placenta 2002;23:392–399.
61 Taricco E, Radaelli T, Rossi G, Nobile de Santis MS, Bulfamante GP, Avagliano L, Cetin I: Effects of gestational diabetes on fetal oxygen and glucose levels in vivo. BJOG 2009; 116:1729–1735.
62 Cetin I, de Santis MS, Taricco E, Radaelli T, Teng C, Ronzoni S, Spada E, Milani S, Pardi G: Maternal and fetal amino acid concentrations in normal pregnancies and in pregnancies with gestational diabetes mellitus. Am J Obstet Gynecol 2005;192:610–617.
63 Magnusson AL, Waterman IJ, Wennergren M, Jansson T, Powell TL: Triglyceride hydrolase activities and expression of fatty acid binding proteins in the human placenta in pregnancies complicated by intrauterine growth restriction and diabetes. J Clin Endocrinol Metab 2004;89:4607–4614.
64 Miozzo M, Simoni G: The role of imprinted genes in fetal growth. Biol Neonate 2002;81: 217–228.
65 Roberts CT, Kind KL, Earl RA, Grant PA, Robinson JS, Sohlstrom A, Owens PC, Owens JA: Circulating insulin-like growth factor (IFG)-1 and IGF binding proteins-1 and -3 and placental development in the guinea pig. Placenta 2002;23:763–770.
66 Sferruzzi-Perri AN, Owens JA, Pringle KG, Robinson JS, Roberts CT: Maternal insulin-like growth factor-I and -II act via different pathways to promote fetal growth. Endocrinology 2006;147:3344–3355.
67 Kniss DA, Shubert PJ, Zimmerman PD, Landon MB, Grabbe SG: Insulin-like growth factors: their regulation of glucose and amino acid transport in placental trophoblast isolated from first-trimester chorionic villi. J Reprod Med 1994;39:249–256.
68 Randhawa R, Cohen P: The role of the insulin-like growth factor system in prenatal growth. Mol Genet Metab 2005;86:84–90.
69 Efstradiadis A: Genetics of mouse growth. Int J Dev Biol 1998;42:955–976.
70 Constância M, Hemberger M, Hughes J, Dean W, Ferguson-Smith A, Fundele R, Stewart F, Kelsey G, Fowden A, Sibley C, Reik W: Placental-specific IGF-II is a major modulator of placental and fetal growth. Nature 2002;417:945–848.
71 Root S, Lagerlöf O, Wennergren M, Powell TL, Jansson T: Regulation of amino acid transporters by glucose and growth factors in cultured primary human trophoblast cells is mediated by mTOR signaling. Am J Physiol Cell Physiol 2009;297:C723–C731.
72 Radaelli T, Cetin I, Boito S, Cozzi V, Taricco M, Alvino G, Iurlaro E, Martinelli A, Pardi G: Fetal oxygen uptake in normal and IUGR pregnancies (abstract OC250). 17th World Congr Ultrasound Obstet Gynecol ISUOG, Florence, October 7–11 2007. Ultrasound Obstet Gynecol 2007;30.
73 Ortega-Senovilla H, Alvino G, Taricco E, Cetin I, Herrera E: Gestational diabetes mellitus impairs the proportion of fatty acids in umbilical arterial but not venous plasma. Diabetes Care 2009;32:120–122.
74 Leunda-Casi A, de Hertogh R, Pampfer S: Decreased expression of fibroblast, growth factor 4 and associated dysregulation of trophoblast differentiation in mouse blastocyst exposed to high D-glucose in vitro. Diabetologia 2001;44:1318–1325.
75 Leunda-Casi A, Genicot G, Donnay I, Pampfer S, de Hertogh R: Increased cell death in mouse blastocysts exposed to high D-glucose in vitro: implication of an antioxidant stress in glucose metabolism. Diabetologia 2002; 45:571–579.
76 Smedts HPM, Rakhshanderhoo M, Verkleij-Hagoort AC, de Vries JHM, Ottenkamp J, Steegers EAP, Steegers-Theunissen RPM: Maternal intake of fat, riboflavin and nicotinamide and the risk of having offspring with congenital heart defects. Eur J Nutr 2008;47:357–365.
77 Vujkovic M, Ocke MC, van der Spek PJ, Yazdanpanah N, Steegers EA, Steegers-Theunissen RPM: Maternal Western dietary patterns and the risk of developing a cleft lip with or without a cleft palate. Obstet Gynecol 2007;110:378–384.
78 Van Eijsden M, Smits LJ, van der Wal MF, Bonsel GJ Association between short interpregnancy intervals and term birth weight: the role of folate depletion. Am J Clin Nutr 2008;88:147–153.
79 Czeizel AE, Tímár L, Sárközi: A dose-dependent effect of folic acid on the prevention of orofacial clefts. Pediatrics 1999;10:e66.
80 Tamura T, Picciano MF: Folate and human reproduction. Am J Clin Nutr 2006;83:993–1016.
81 Zhou LM, Yang WW, Hua JZ, Deng CQ, Tao X, Stoltzfus RJ: Relation of hemoglobin measured at different times in pregnancy to preterm birth and low birth weight in Shanghai, China. Am J Epidemiol 1998;148:998–1006.
82 Verkleij-Hagoort AC, de Vries JH, Ursem NT, de Jonge R, Hop WC, Steegers-Theunissen RP: Dietary intake of B vitamins in mothers born a child with a congenital heart defect. Eur J Nutr 2006;45:478–486.
83 Cattanach BM, Peters J, Ball S, Rasberry C: Two imprinted gene mutations: three phenotypes. Hum Mol Genet 2000;9:2263–2273.
84 Coan PM, Burton GJ Ferguson-Smith AC: Imprinted genes in the placenta – a review. Placenta 2005; 26(supplement A):S10–S20.
85 Bressan FF, De Bem THC, Perecin F, Lopes FL, Ambrosio CE, Meirelles FV, Miglino MA: Unearthing the roles of imprinted genes in the placenta. Placenta 2009;30:823–834.

Annales Nestlé

Ann Nestlé [Engl] 2010;68:17–28
DOI: 10.1159/000298780

Weight Gain during Pregnancy: Importance for Maternal and Child Health

Sharon J. Herring[a] Emily Oken[b]

[a]Center for Obesity Research and Education, Temple University School of Medicine, Philadelphia, Pa., and
[b]Obesity Prevention Program, Department of Population Medicine, Harvard Medical School and Harvard Pilgrim Health Care, Boston, Mass., USA

Key Words
Gestational weight gain · Pregnancy · Maternal health · Child health · Postpartum · Preterm birth · Fetal growth · Obesity

Abstract
Gestational weight gain is a strong predictor of short- and long-term health outcomes for both childbearing women and their offspring. Epidemiologic studies have found that higher maternal gestational weight gains are associated with abnormalities in maternal prenatal glycemia, hypertensive disorders of pregnancy and delivery complications, along with an increased risk of postpartum weight retention, incident obesity and adverse cardiometabolic sequelae in mothers by midlife. Additionally, observational data have linked greater gestational weight gains to increased fetal growth and later childhood obesity. Associations of gestational weight gain with preterm birth and infant mortality may be U-shaped, such that the risks are increased with both low and high gains. In an attempt to optimize both maternal and child outcomes, the Institute of Medicine revised gestational weight gain guidelines in 2009, recommending smaller gains for women with higher prepregnancy body mass indices, particularly for women entering pregnancy with a body mass index of at least 30. However, it is as of yet unclear if these new recommendations will lead to improvements in the proportions of women gaining recommended amounts, and in maternal and child health. As fewer than one third of mothers currently gain within the ranges recommended by the Institute of Medicine, interventions to help mothers achieve healthy gestational weight gains are of critical public health importance.

Introduction

Gestational weight gain is a strong predictor of infant outcomes at birth [1]. It is well established that gestational weight gain is directly associated with intrauterine growth, and thus, infants born to women who gain more weight during pregnancy are less likely to be born small for gestational age or at low birth weight [1, 2]. Both very low and very high gestational weight gains are associated with an increased risk of preterm birth and infant death

KARGER

Fax +41 61 306 12 34
E-Mail karger@karger.ch
www.karger.com

0517–8606/10/0681–0017$26.00/0

Accessible online at:
www.karger.com/ane

Sharon J. Herring, MD
Center for Obesity Research and Education
Temple University School of Medicine, 3223 N. Broad Street, Suite 175
Philadelphia, PA 19140 (USA)
Tel. +1 215 707 2234, Fax +1 215 707 6475, E-Mail Sharon.Herring@temple.edu

Table 1. Total weight gains and rates of weight gain recommended for women with singleton pregnancies in the 2009 IOM guidelines

Prepregnancy weight status (body mass index category)	Recommended total weight gain ranges, kg	Recommended rates of weight gain in the 2nd and 3rd trimesters[1] kg/week
Underweight (<18.5)	12.5–18	0.51 (0.44–0.58)
Normal (18.5–24.9)	11.5–16	0.42 (0.35–0.50)
Overweight (25–29.9)	7–11.5	0.28 (0.23–0.33)
Obese (≥30)	5–9	0.22 (0.17–0.27)

Adapted from IOM [1].
[1] Calculations assume a weight gain of 0.5–2 kg in the first trimester.

[3]. In an attempt to improve neonatal outcomes, recommendations for weight gain during pregnancy have increased since the early part of the 20th century, from 7 kg in the 1930s to 11.5–16 kg for normal weight-women in 1990 [4]. Actual gestational weight gains have been increasing in excess of the guidelines [5], and in recent years, nearly half of women in the USA gained more than recommended [6].

However, more weight gain may not always be better. Recent studies have highlighted some of the negative health outcomes associated with greater gains during pregnancy [3], including delivery complications [7], childhood overweight [8–10] and higher postpartum weight retention, which predisposes to later risk of obesity in the mother [6, 11].

In an attempt to optimize both maternal and child outcomes, in 2009 the United States Institute of Medicine (IOM) revised gestational weight gain guidelines for the first time since 1990 (table 1) [1]. These guidelines recommend smaller gains for women with higher prepregnancy body mass indices (BMI), particularly for women entering pregnancy with a BMI of at least 30. Given these more stringent recommendations, the proportion of women gaining above the suggested levels is likely to increase, unless successful interventions can interrupt trends toward higher gains.

In this article we review the physiology and sociodemographic predictors of gestational weight gain. We summarize the evidence underlying the 2009 IOM gestational weight gain guidelines [1, 3], as well as more recent studies not incorporated into the guidelines. We discuss mechanisms by which maternal weight gain during pregnancy influences maternal and child health outcomes, incorporating data from human trials and animal studies. Finally, we discuss strategies to help mothers achieve healthy pregnancy weight gains.

Components of Gestational Weight Gain

The weight gained in a normal pregnancy includes biologic processes designed to foster fetal growth [12]. Although women vary in the composition of the weight they gain during pregnancy, a general picture can be drawn. Approximately 25–30% of the weight gain resides in the fetus, 30–40% resides in maternal reproductive tissues, placenta, fluid and blood, and about 30% is made up of maternal fat stores [1]. In early pregnancy, normal-weight women (prepregnancy BMI <25) deposit fat in their hips, back and upper thighs, which is thought to be important as a caloric reserve for late pregnancy and lactation [12]. Insulin secretion and sensitivity rise, favoring increased lipogenesis and fat accumulation, in preparation for the increased energy needs of the growing fetus [13]. However, in obese women (prepregnancy BMI ≥30), peripheral insulin sensitivity declines, and little or no increased fat is accrued in early pregnancy, perhaps due to a reduced need for additional caloric reserves [14]. By late pregnancy, insulin resistance increases among all mothers (although it is more pronounced in obese women), a normal physiologic adaptation that shifts maternal energy metabolism from carbohydrate to lipid oxidation and thus spares glucose for the fetus [15].

The pattern of gestational weight gain is most commonly described as sigmoidal, with the majority of weight gained in the 2nd and early 3rd trimesters of pregnancy

[1]. Across studies published in the USA since 1985, total pregnancy weight gains of normal-weight adult women giving birth to healthy term infants ranged from a low of 10.0 kg to a high of 16.7 kg, while lower gestational weight gains have been described among obese (mean gain = 11 kg) and very obese (mean gain = 9 kg) women [1].

Who Is at the Greatest Risk of Under- or Over-Gain in Pregnancy?

A complex interplay among biological, psychological and social contextual factors influences the amount of weight a woman gains in pregnancy. Despite the consistent inverse relationship observed between total gestational weight gain and pregravid BMI category, overweight and obese women are nearly 2 times more likely to exceed 1990 IOM recommended gains compared to normal-weight women [16, 17]. Underweight women, on the other hand, are more likely to gain below 1990 IOM recommendations [16]. Additionally, multiparity, smoking during pregnancy, older age and being of low income, black or Hispanic race/ethnicity, unmarried status and limited education are associated with inadequate gain [1, 18, 19]. A number of the same sociodemographic characteristics have emerged as risk factors for gaining above the IOM recommendations. For example, among a sample of 622 predominately white women living in New York State, Olson et al. [20] found that those with household incomes <185% of the US federal poverty line were 2.5 times more likely to gain excessively in pregnancy than the women with higher incomes. Lederman et al. [21] found that over two thirds of low-income Black women in New York City gained more than recommended by the IOM, and 100% of the overweight and obese women experienced excessive gain.

However, some risk factors have been understudied. Although dietary intake, physical inactivity, television viewing and insufficient sleep are associated with weight gain in nonpregnant women and men [22–24], limited data exist on these factors during pregnancy. The contributions of specific genes and sequence variants to higher and lower gestational weight gains are also still unclear. A better understanding of the characteristics of women at the highest risk of inadequate and excessive weight gain is critical in order to aggressively target these mothers in interventions aimed at achieving healthy pregnancy weight gains, and thus lead to improvements in the maternal and child outcomes described in this review.

Gestational Weight Gain and Maternal Health Outcomes

Maternal Health Outcomes during Pregnancy

Glucose Metabolism

Gestational diabetes mellitus (GDM) is defined as glucose intolerance initially diagnosed during pregnancy. In about 7% of women, the acceleration of insulin resistance in late pregnancy is accompanied by insufficient pancreatic β-cell insulin secretion, and GDM ensues [15, 25]. Both GDM and more moderate states of abnormal glucose tolerance in pregnancy are associated with an increase in perinatal complications [26] and later development of type 2 diabetes in both mother and child [27, 28].

It is plausible that greater gestational weight gains would increase the risk of abnormal glucose tolerance in pregnancy. Weight gain and obesity promote incident diabetes in nonpregnant individuals, as excess adiposity results in insulin resistance and ultimately in pancreatic β-cell exhaustion [29, 30]. Maternal weight entering pregnancy is among the strongest identified predictors for the development of GDM [31, 32]. Furthermore, interpregnancy weight gain predicts the risk of GDM in a subsequent pregnancy [33].

Most early studies examining associations of gestational weight gain with risk of GDM were limited in that they assessed total gestational weight gain [3]. Diagnosis of GDM, which generally occurs when routine glycemic screening is administered at 24–28 weeks' gestation, may influence subsequent weight gain. A few recent studies have examined associations of weight gain prior to glycemic screening with risk of abnormal glucose tolerance. In a study of women enrolled in the Pregnancy, Infancy and Nutrition cohort, Saldana et al. [34] found a 2-fold increased risk of impaired glucose tolerance (a moderate state of abnormal glucose tolerance in pregnancy) among overweight women who gained weight at a rate higher than recommended by the IOM prior to glycemic screening. However, this measure of gestational weight gain was not related to any increase in risk of GDM, and no associations were evident in normal-weight or obese mothers. We found similar results among women in the Project Viva cohort (fig. 1), although there was no interaction with prepregnancy BMI [35]. Another recent cohort study also revealed a direct relationship of weight gain prior to glycemic screening in excess of IOM guidelines with glucose intolerance, although these findings were limited to Hispanic women with a BMI of at least 35 [36].

Evidence that the association between higher gestational weight gain and hyperglycemia may be causal

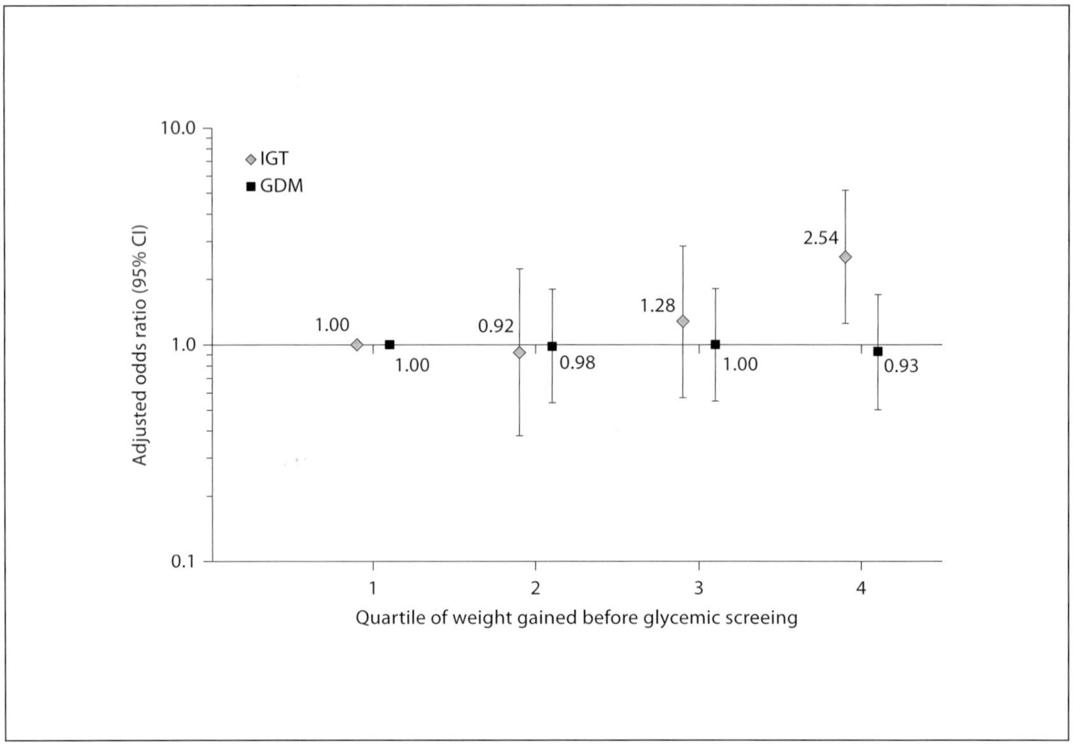

Fig. 1. Odds of developing impaired glucose tolerance (IGT) in pregnancy or GDM by quartile of gestational weight gained before glycemic screening, Project Viva, 1999–2002. Estimates adjusted for gestational age at glycemic screening, age, race/ethnicity, prepregnancy BMI category and history of gestational diabetes (from Herring et al. [35]).

comes from a recent clinical trial. Among 50 obese Danish women enrolled in a dietary counseling intervention in early pregnancy, Wolff et al. [37] reported lower weight gain throughout pregnancy, a 20% reduction in serum insulin levels at 27 weeks' gestation and an 8% reduction in fasting blood glucose at 36 weeks' gestation compared with women who did not receive the intervention. The intervention women did not experience a reduction in risk of GDM, however, suggesting that changes in weight during pregnancy may have a greater impact on more moderate levels of glucose intolerance.

Overall, the available data suggest a direct relationship between gestational weight gain during the first 2 trimesters of pregnancy and moderate levels of abnormal glucose tolerance at glycemic screening. However, no convincing evidence indicates that lower weight gains are associated with lower risk of developing GDM. Whether the absence of a relationship between weight gain and GDM is related to other, unmeasured factors, such as β-cell exhaustion or pregnancy-specific alterations in insulin resistance [38, 39], that predispose women to GDM independent of weight-related changes, is still unclear. It is possible that the timing or pattern of metabolic changes responsible for frank GDM is different from those predicting moderate states of glucose intolerance in pregnancy [40, 41].

Hypertensive Disorders

Complicating 6–8% of pregnancies, hypertensive disorders are common medical problems encountered during pregnancy that remain a leading source of maternal and fetal morbidity [42]. Hypertensive disorders during pregnancy include gestational hypertension (new-onset, nonproteinuric hypertension first observed after 20 weeks' gestation) and preeclampsia (new-onset hypertension with proteinuria and edema after 20 weeks of gestation) [42]. Most established risk factors for gestational hypertension or preeclampsia, including maternal age, race/ethnicity, parity, and previous hypertension or preeclampsia, are not modifiable [43]. During the past 2 decades, a number of studies have examined whether maternal weight gain in pregnancy might influence the risk of pregnancy-induced hypertension, given the strong association between weight gain and high blood pressure in nonpregnant adults [44].

The majority of epidemiologic studies have reported a direct relationship between greater weight gain in pregnancy and the onset of gestational hypertension and/or preeclampsia [45–54]. Additionally, weight gain within or below IOM-recommended ranges may be protective against the onset of hypertensive disorders during pregnancy. A large prospective cohort study from Sweden found that gains of <8 kg were associated with reduced odds of developing preeclampsia for women in all pregravid BMI categories, compared to a reference gain of 8–16 kg [47]. Similarly, Kiel et al. [48] found a decreased risk of preeclampsia among obese women gaining <7 kg. Since edema is one of the diagnostic criteria for preeclampsia, however, it is still unclear whether the observed association is truly related to excess gain in body fat or whether it is just a by-product of excess fluid retention.

Delivery Complications

Two systematic reviews that included data from >500,000 pregnancies in 21 studies have found a consistent dose-response relationship between pregnancy weight gain and cesarean delivery [3, 4]. Weight gains within or below IOM-recommended ranges may be protective against cesarean delivery [48]. In addition, recent data suggest that weight gains in excess of IOM recommendations lead to increased odds of other delivery complications, including failed induction and cephalopelvic disproportion, compared to gains within the recommended range, in women of all prepregnancy BMI categories [46, 47, 49].

Postpartum and Long-Term Maternal Health

Postpartum Weight Retention, Obesity Risk and Cardiometabolic Sequelae

In observational epidemiologic studies, gestational weight gain is the strongest predictor of maternal weight change from prepregnancy through 18 months postpartum, accounting for 20–35% of the variability in weight change [11, 55–59]. In addition to the total amount of weight gain, the pattern of gain may influence weight retention. Kleinman et al. [60] found that weight gains earlier in pregnancy were more predictive of weight retention at 6 months postpartum compared with the same amount of gain accrued later in pregnancy.

Postpartum weight retention appears particularly likely among Black women and those who enter pregnancy overweight or obese [11, 59, 61]. Among all women, postpartum weight retention is associated with short- and long-term risk of overweight. Approximately 6–14% of women develop overweight within 1 year after delivery [62]. Additionally, Linne et al. [63] reported that nearly 44% of women who were normal weight entering pregnancy but retained significant amounts of weight (approximately 4.8 kg) at 12 months postpartum became overweight 15 years later.

Compared with weight gain during other periods, excess weight gain associated with childbearing appears to be particularly harmful, as it is deposited in central rather than peripheral sites [64], it is associated with reductions in HDL cholesterol [65] and with an increased risk of metabolic syndrome by midlife [66]. One mechanism for the persistent cardiometabolic derangements of pregnancy may be increases in intra-abdominal (visceral) adiposity. A 5-year longitudinal study found a 40% increase in visceral fat from preconception to postpartum versus a 14% increase among nonparous women followed for the same amount of time [67]. Intra-abdominal adipose tissue is associated with obesity-related insulin resistance, production of adipocytokines that regulate insulin sensitivity and dyslipidemia [30, 68]. Whether this metabolic risk is minimized by achieving guideline-recommended gestational weight gains and postpartum weight loss, is still unclear; interventions are needed to test whether mothers' short- and long-term metabolic status improves.

In summary, gestational weight gain is associated with several short- and longer-term maternal health outcomes. For all of these maternal outcomes, less gain is better. In contrast, as we review below, greater gestational weight gain is associated with improvements in some infant health outcomes, but increased risk for others.

Gestational Weight Gain and Child Health Outcomes

Gestational Weight Gain and Infant Health

Fetal Growth

The direct association between maternal gestational weight gain and infant weight at birth has been recognized for decades and was one of the primary drivers for the IOM to generate recommendations for higher weight gains in 1990 [69]. In a recent evidence review of publications from 1990 through 2007, Viswanathan et al. [3] found moderate to strong evidence suggesting an association of weight gain below IOM recommendations with low birth weight and small for gestational age (SGA) births, and strong evidence for the relationship between weight gain above IOM recommendations and high birth weight, macrosomia and large for gestational age (LGA) births [70].

Most studies have examined weight, or weight for gestational age, as infant outcomes. However, weight tends to track with linear growth. Some studies have found similar associations between maternal weight gain and measures of infant weight adjusted for length [71]. In one study, weight gain in midpregnancy predicted infant length as well as weight at birth [72]. In addition, weight comprises both fat and lean mass. If higher weight gain promotes greater increase in lean body mass, that may be desirable, but if higher weight gain predicts only gain in fat mass, then that may be a less favorable result. Data regarding direct measures of adiposity are extremely limited [73].

Associations of gestational weight gain with higher infant weight at birth are generally independent of maternal prepregnancy BMI, although some evidence suggests that the associations may be particularly strong among women who are normal weight or underweight entering pregnancy. Among women who are obese, gestational weight gain is a less strong predictor of fetal growth [74]. Although some groups of mothers are at greater risk of having a SGA infant, such as mothers who are black, teenagers, of short stature or smoke during pregnancy, higher gains do not appear to equalize risks for these mothers [75].

Most evidence linking gestational weight gain with fetal growth comes from observational studies. As observational research cannot determine causality, it is possible that other factors underlie the relationship between greater maternal and infant weight gains. Most obviously, since the weight gained by the mother includes that gained by the infant, higher birth weight results in greater total gestational weight gain. However, associations persist in studies that have used net gestational weight gain (i.e. birth weight subtracted from total weight gain) as an exposure [76]. In addition, it is possible that shared genes underlie greater maternal and fetal weight gain. However, in a study of 90 pairs of siblings, greater gestational weight gain was associated with higher birth weight on a within-mother analysis [77]. Furthermore, mean birth weight among term infants increased during the second half of the 20th century in the USA, Canada and other countries, a trend not likely to be attributable to shifts in genes but that appeared to be caused by parallel increases in gestational weight gain and other maternal characteristics [78–80].

Thus, it is likely that associations of higher gestational weight gains with greater fetal growth are causal. Moderate gains are recommended to minimize the risk of the child being either small for gestational age or large for gestational age.

Preterm Birth and Infant Mortality

In their recent evidence review, Viswanathan et al. [3] found strong evidence suggesting that both low and high weight gains result in an increased risk of premature birth. Eight of 9 studies reported at least 1 significant association between low gestational weight gain and preterm birth; 4 of 5 studies focused on high gestational weight gain (as defined in each study) reported at least 1 significant association between gestational weight gain and preterm birth [3]. Overall, the majority of studies found a consistent effect of low gestational weight gain on preterm birth and a less consistent effect of high gestational weight gain on preterm birth. The association for low gestational weight gain holds whether total weight gain or rate of weight gain is used as the relevant exposure of interest.

Viswanathan et al. [3] summarized 3 studies that looked at the association between maternal weight gain and infant mortality. None of them was rated as good quality. Overall, these studies suggest a protective effect of gestational weight gain on perinatal mortality but not on stillbirth. In more recent publication data from the US National Maternal and Infant Health Survey, maternal prepregnancy obesity as well as very low and very high rates of weight gain were each associated with infant death. For example, compared with normal-weight women who gained 0.30–0.44 kg/week, obese women who gained <0.15 kg/week had an adjusted odds ratio of infant death of 1.75 (95% CI = 1.28–2.39), and obese women who gained ≥0.45 kg/week had an odds ratio of 2.87 (95% CI = 1.98–4.16).

Thus, gestational weight gain appears to have a U-shaped relationship with both preterm birth and infant death. Similar to the fetal growth outcomes, moderate gains are optimal.

Gestational Weight Gain and Longer-Term Child Health

Childhood Weight Status and Risk of Obesity

A number of observational epidemiologic studies have found that higher maternal gestational weight gain is associated with higher weight in childhood [8–10], adoles-

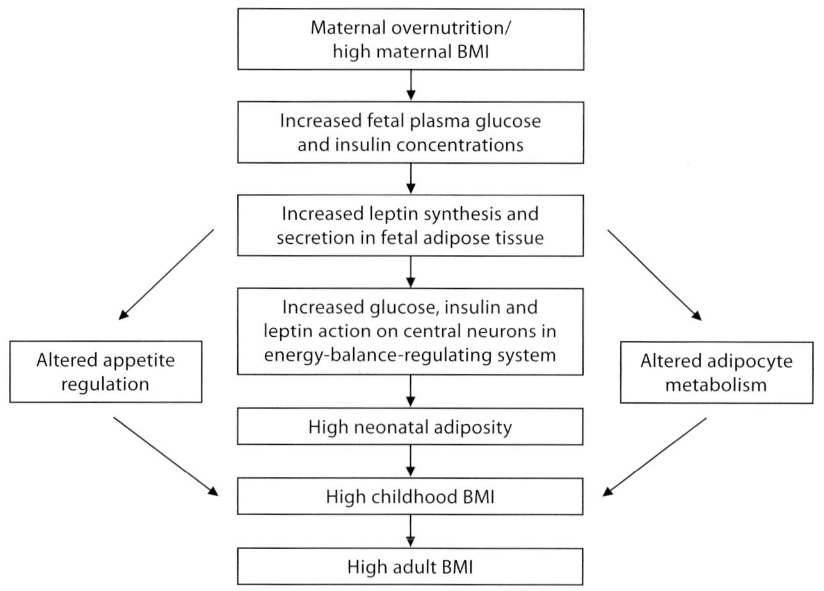

Fig. 2. Potential pathways explaining the relationship between maternal nutrition and offspring obesity (from McMillen et al. [90]).

cence [81, 82] and adulthood [83, 84]. One found an association of higher gestational weight gain with increased risk of early-onset, but not late-onset, childhood obesity [85]. However, a direct association between higher gestational weight gain and child adiposity has not been found in all studies [86, 87].

Some studies have reported a U- or J-shaped association, with greater overweight risks with the lowest maternal gains, especially in women with lower prepregnancy BMI [83]. However, in a recent study we observed an apparent U-shaped relationship between gestational weight gain and attained offspring weight in adolescence, which became linear after adjustment for maternal prepregnancy BMI [82]. This shift is derived from the fact that women who enter pregnancy at a higher weight tend to gain less weight during pregnancy and highlights the importance of considering both prepregnancy weight and gestational weight gain.

It is unclear whether associations of gestational weight gain with child weight vary by maternal prepregnancy weight. Some studies found stronger associations among overweight and obese mothers [8], some observed somewhat stronger relationships among underweight mothers [9, 88], one found an effect only among mothers currently normal weight but not overweight [89], and others reported no evidence for effect modification by maternal BMI [10, 82].

How might excess weight gain during pregnancy have a persistent influence on offspring weight and related cardiometabolic risk? Shared genes and behaviors certainly explain part of the risk. In addition, maternal overnutrition appears to have a direct influence on several aspects of offspring physiology, including appetite, metabolism and activity levels (fig. 2) [90]. Offspring of overfed rat dams have reduced energy expenditure [91, 92] and a greater taste for junk food [93], as do human children of obese mothers [94, 95]. Lambs of overfed ewes have changes in the central appetite regulatory system, altered gene expression in adipose tissue and increased expression of leptin [96–98]. Maternal overnutrition may result in increased fetal adipose tissue deposition [99]. Since adipocyte number appears to be set in the first years of life [100], excess fat formed in early life may result in lifelong excess adiposity. Maternal prenatal overnutrition may also influence the fetal epigenome, thereby affecting the expression of genes that direct the accumulation of body fat or related metabolism [101–103].

Other Child Outcomes

If higher gestational weight gains result in child obesity, it is plausible that they would also be associated with the adverse sequelae of obesity. We have found that children whose mothers gained excess weight during pregnancy had higher blood pressure [8] and poorer cognitive test scores [104] at age 3 years. To date, few studies have examined child outcomes other than weight or have information on offspring in later life.

Balancing the Risks and Benefits of Too Much or Too Little Gestational Weight Gain

Overall, too much or too little weight gain in pregnancy appears to have a profound impact on the health of mothers and their children. While higher amounts of weight gain generally seem to be harmful for both maternal short- and longer-term health outcomes after childbirth, the same is not true for infants. Determining optimal gestational weight gain is complicated by the fact that associations with outcomes may differ not only in strength and direction but also in seriousness. In 2009, we used data from the Project Viva cohort to determine the most favorable amount of weight gain considering 5 short- and longer-term outcomes: short for gestational age, large for gestational age, preterm delivery, substantial maternal postpartum weight retention and child obesity [74]. We found that lowest-risk gestational weight gains were within 1990 recommended ranges for women who were normal weight entering pregnancy but were lower than the recommendations for overweight and obese women [74]. In all models, the lowest predicted prevalence of adverse outcomes for obese women occurred with weight loss. Our data suggest that more research is needed to determine optimal gain in mothers, taking into account the risks and benefits of too little and too much gain, particularly for mothers who begin pregnancy overweight and obese. While the 2009 IOM guidelines recommend somewhat smaller weight gains for obese mothers compared with 1990 guidelines, it is still unclear whether even greater weight restriction among obese mothers, or no weight gain at all, will achieve the best maternal and child outcomes.

Strategies to Achieve Healthy Pregnancy Weight Gains

Despite continued debate over the optimal range of gestational weight gain for overweight and obese mothers, too few mothers of all pregravid BMI categories gain within the recommended ranges [6]. Thus, a big question remains: how can we help more mothers achieve recommended gestational weight gains? Because pregnant women have frequent interactions with the health care system, obstetric clinicians are uniquely positioned to address weight gain with their pregnant patients. In fact, data suggest that medically advised and actual pregnancy weight gains are strongly correlated [105, 106]. Several interventions to promote recommended gestational weight gain have included clinician advice as one component of the intervention [107–110]. However, these interventions have generally not been successful in improving the proportion of women gaining within recommended limits [107] or were successful only in a subset of women [108].

Many obstetric clinicians are not providing their patients with any guidance regarding the appropriate amount of gestational weight gain. In a national survey, only 58% of obstetrician-gynecologists reported counseling their pregnant patients about weight gain during pregnancy 'most of the time', and even fewer (35.7%) modified their recommendations based on their patients' prepregnancy BMI [111]. Further, the obstetric providers who do advise their patients may not be recommending gestational weight gain ranges concordant with IOM guidelines. In a 2007–2008 survey of 58 obstetric providers in Massachusetts, we found that provider gestational weight gain recommendations were generally discordant with 1990 IOM guidelines [112]. Our data suggest a need for better dissemination of recommended gains to obstetric providers, to arm them with the correct information for advising their pregnant patients.

In addition to recommending the right amounts of gain, clinicians may also need to counsel women regarding how to achieve these recommended gains. The 2009 IOM report does not provide any detailed guidance concerning specific components of diet or other behaviors to achieve healthy gains. Many clinicians indicate that they do not have sufficient time or knowledge to counsel women regarding weight-related behaviors [112]. Further, obstetricians may not be comfortable discussing weight-related behaviors with their patients or may feel that their advice does not influence their patients in making changes [112]. Specially trained ancillary staff, including dieticians, health coaches and public health nurses, may be helpful adjuncts in delivering nutrition and healthy weight gain messages to pregnant mothers [37, 113–115]. For example, in 2008, Wolff et al. [37] randomized 50 obese pregnant women in Denmark to either ten 1-hour dietary consultations with a trained dietician or to usual care. The women in the intervention group successfully limited their energy intake and restricted their total gestational weight gain to an average of 6.6 kg compared to 13.3 kg in the control group. However, the small sample size and different healthcare settings have limited the widespread adoption of these intervention strategies to date.

Few interventions have focused on minority mothers, who are at high risk of both undernutrition and overgain. Additionally, no studies have followed both mothers and their children into the postpartum period, to evaluate the effect of interventions on longer-term maternal and child health outcomes. More research is needed to help all women achieve healthy pregnancy weight and behaviors, assessing both short- and longer-term health outcomes.

In summary, efforts to help mothers gain within IOM-recommended ranges in pregnancy are critical to keeping mothers and their children healthy. These efforts are also likely to be economical, as a single intervention could benefit the mother, her child, future pregnancies and subsequent generations. Ongoing and planned research will provide greater guidance in the coming years regarding the best way to support women in achieving optimal gains.

References

1 Institute of Medicine: Weight Gain During Pregnancy: Reexamining the Guidelines. Washington, National Academy Press, 2009.

2 Luke B, Hediger ML, Scholl TO: Point of diminishing returns: when does gestational weight gain cease benefiting birth weight and begin adding to maternal obesity? J Matern Fetal Med 1996;5:168–173.

3 Viswanathan M, Siega-Riz AM, Moos MK, Deierlein A, Mumford S, Knaack J, Thieda P, Lux LJ, Lohr KN: Outcomes of maternal weight gain. Evid Rep Technol Assess 2008: 1–223.

4 Abrams B, Altman SL, Pickett KE: Pregnancy weight gain: still controversial. Am J Clin Nutr 2000;71:1233S–1241S.

5 Helms E, Coulson CC, Galvin SL: Trends in weight gain during pregnancy: a population study across 16 years in North Carolina. Am J Obstet Gynecol 2006;194:e32–e34.

6 Olson CM: Achieving a healthy weight gain during pregnancy. Annu Rev Nutr 2008;28: 411–423.

7 Catalano PM: Management of obesity in pregnancy. Obstet Gynecol 2007;109:419–433.

8 Olson CM, Strawderman MS, Dennison BA: Maternal weight gain during pregnancy and child weight at age 3 years. Matern Child Health J 2009;13:839–846.

9 Wrotniak BH, Shults J, Butts S, Stettler N: Gestational weight gain and risk of overweight in the offspring at age 7 years in a multicenter, multiethnic cohort study. Am J Clin Nutr 2008;87:1818–1824.

10 Oken E, Taveras EM, Kleinman KP, Rich-Edwards JW, Gillman MW: Gestational weight gain and child adiposity at age 3 years. Am J Obste Gynecol 2007;196:322. e321–e328.

11 Gunderson EP, Abrams B: Epidemiology of gestational weight gain and body weight changes after pregnancy. Epidemiol Rev 2000;22:261–274.

12 Worthington-Roberts BS, Williams SR: Nutrition throughout the Life Cycle, ed 3. St Louis, Mosby, 1996.

13 Lain KY, Catalano PM: Metabolic changes in pregnancy. Clin Obstet Gynecol 2007;50: 938–948.

14 Lang K, King J: Doctoral dissertation. Berkeley, University of California, 2009.

15 Boden G: Fuel metabolism in pregnancy and in gestational diabetes mellitus. Obstet Gynecol Clin North Am 1996;23:1–10.

16 Wells CS, Schwalberg R, Noonan G, Gabor V: Factors influencing inadequate and excessive weight gain in pregnancy: Colorado, 2000–2002. Matern Child Health J 2006;10: 55–62.

17 Brawarsky P, Stotland NE, Jackson RA, Fuentes-Afflick E, Escobar GJ, Rubashkin N, Haas JS: Pre-pregnancy and pregnancy-related factors and the risk of excessive or inadequate gestational weight gain. Int J Gynaecol Obstet 2005;91:125–131.

18 Hickey CA, Cliver SP, McNeal SF, Hoffman HJ, Goldenberg RL: Prenatal weight gain patterns and spontaneous preterm birth among nonobese black and white women. Obstet Gynecol 1995;85:909–914.

19 Siega-Riz AM, Hobel CJ: Predictors of poor maternal weight gain from baseline anthropometric, psychosocial, and demographic information in a Hispanic population. J Am Diet Assoc 1997;97:1264–1268.

20 Olson CM, Strawderman MS: Modifiable behavioral factors in a biopsychosocial model predict inadequate and excessive gestational weight gain. J American Diet Assoc 2003; 103:48–54.

21 Lederman SA, Alfasi G, Deckelbaum RJ: Pregnancy-associated obesity in black women in New York City. Matern Child Health J 2002;6:37–42.

22 Hu FB: Obesity Epidemiology. New York, Oxford University Press, 2008.

23 Oken E, Taveras EM, Popoola FA, Rich-Edwards JW, Gillman MW: Television, walking, and diet: associations with postpartum weight retention. Am J Prevent Med 2007;32: 305–311.

24 Gunderson EP, Rifas-Shiman SL, Oken E, Rich-Edwards JW, Kleinman KP, Taveras EM, Gillman MW: Association of fewer hours of sleep at 6 months postpartum with substantial weight retention at 1 year postpartum. Am J Epidemiol 2008;167:178–187.

25 American Diabetes Association: Standards of medical care in diabetes. Diabetes Care 2008;31:S13–S54.
26 Metzger BE, Lowe LP, Dyer AR, Trimble ER, Chaovarindr U, Coustan DR, Hadden DR, McCance DR, Hod M, McIntyre HD, Oats JJN, Persson B, Rogers MS, Sacks DA, HAPO study cooperative research group: Hyperglycemia and adverse pregnancy outcomes. N Engl J Med 2008;358:1991–2002.
27 Hillier TA, Pedula KL, Schmidt MM, Mullen JA, Charles M-A, Pettitt DJ: Childhood obesity and metabolic imprinting: the ongoing effects of maternal hyperglycemia. Diabetes Care 2007;30:2287–2292.
28 Retnakaran R, Qi Y, Sermer M, Connelly PW, Hanley AJ, Zinman B: Glucose intolerance in pregnancy and future risk of pre-diabetes or diabetes. Diabetes Care 2008;31:2026–2031.
29 Reaven GM: Insulin resistance and human disease: a short history. J Basic Clin Physiol Pharmacol 1998;9:387–406.
30 Rondinone CM: Adipocyte-derived hormones, cytokines, and mediators. Endocrine 2006;29:81–90.
31 Solomon CG, Willett WC, Carey VJ, Rich-Edwards J, Hunter DJ, Colditz GA, Stampfer MJ, Speizer FE, Spiegelman D, Manson JE: A prospective study of pregravid determinants of gestational diabetes mellitus. JAMA 1997;278:1078–1083.
32 Chu SY, Callaghan WM, Kim SY, Schmid CH, Lau J, England LJ, Dietz PM: Maternal obesity and risk of gestational diabetes mellitus. Diabetes Care 2007;30:2070–2076.
33 Villamor E, Cnattingius S: Interpregnancy weight change and risk of adverse pregnancy outcomes: a population-based study. Lancet 2006;368:1164–1167.
34 Saldana TM, Siega-Riz AM, Adair LS, Suchindran C: The relationship between pregnancy weight gain and glucose tolerance status among black and white women in central North Carolina. Am J Obstet Gynecol 2006;195:1629–1635.
35 Herring SJ, Oken E, Rifas-Shiman SL, Rich-Edwards JW, Stuebe AM, Kleinman KP, Gillman MW: Weight gain in pregnancy and risk of maternal hyperglycemia. Am J Obstet Gynecol 2009;201:61.e61–e67.
36 Tovar A, Must A, Bermudez O, Hyatt R, Chasan-Taber L: The impact of gestational weight gain and diet on abnormal glucose tolerance during pregnancy in Hispanic women. Matern Child Health J 2009;13:520–530.
37 Wolff S, Legarth J, Vangsgaard K, Toubro S, Astrup A: A randomized trial of the effects of dietary counseling on gestational weight gain and glucose metabolism in obese pregnant women. Int J Obes (Lond) 2008;32:495–501.
38 Kahn SE: Clinical review 135: the importance of β-cell failure in the development and progression of type 2 diabetes. J Clin Endocrinol Metab 2001;86:4047–4058.
39 Buchanan TA: Pancreatic B-cell defects in gestational diabetes: implications for the pathogenesis and prevention of type 2 diabetes. J Clin Endocrinol Metab 2001;86:989–993.
40 Kieffer EC, Tabaei BP, Carman WJ, Nolan GH, Guzman JR, Herman WH: The influence of maternal weight and glucose tolerance on infant birth weight in Latino mother-infant pairs. Am J Public Health 2006;96:2201–2208.
41 Retnakaran R, Zinman B, Connelly PW, Sermer M, Hanley AJ: Impaired glucose tolerance of pregnancy is a heterogeneous metabolic disorder as defined by the glycemic response to the oral glucose tolerance test. Diabetes Care 2006;29:57–62.
42 Report of the National High Blood Pressure Education Program Working Group on High Blood Pressure in Pregnancy. Am J Obstet Gynecol 2000;183:S1–S22.
43 Lain KY, Roberts JM: Contemporary concepts of the pathogenesis and management of preeclampsia. JAMA 2002;287:3183–3186.
44 NHLBI Obesity Education Initiative Expert Panel on the Identification, Evaluation, and Treatment of Overweight and Obesity in Adults: Clinical Guidelines on the Identification, Evaluation and Treatment of Overweight and Obesity in Adults. Bethesda, National Heart, Lung and Blood Institute, NIH, 1998.
45 Brennand EA, Dannenbaum D, Willows ND: Pregnancy outcomes of first nations women in relation to pregravid weight and pregnancy weight gain. J Obstet Gynaecol Can 2005;27:936–944.
46 Thorsdottir I, Torfadottir JE, Birgisdottir BE, Geirsson RT: Weight gain in women of normal weight before pregnancy: complications in pregnancy or delivery and birth outcome. Obstet Gynecol 2002;99:799–806.
47 Cedergren M: Effects of gestational weight gain and body mass index on obstetric outcome in Sweden. Int J Gynaecol Obstet 2006;93:269–274.
48 Kiel DW, Dodson EA, Artal R, Boehmer TK, Leet TL: Gestational weight gain and pregnancy outcomes in obese women: how much is enough? Obstet Gynecol 2007;110:752–758.
49 DeVader SR, Neeley HL, Myles TD, Leet TL: Evaluation of gestational weight gain guidelines for women with normal prepregnancy body mass index. Obstet Gynecol 2007;110:745–751.
50 Kabiru W, Raynor BD: Obstetric outcomes associated with increase in BMI category during pregnancy. Am J Obstet Gynecol 2004;191:928–932.
51 Edwards LE, Hellerstedt WL, Alton IR, Story M, Himes JH: Pregnancy complications and birth outcomes in obese and normal-weight women: effects of gestational weight change. Obstet Gynecol 1996;87:389–394.
52 Jensen DM, Ovesen P, Beck-Nielsen H, Molsted-Pedersen L, Sorensen B, Vinter C, Damm P: Gestational weight gain and pregnancy outcomes in 481 obese glucose-tolerant women. Diabetes Care 2005;28:2118–2122.
53 Ogunyemi D, Hullett S, Leeper J, Risk A: Prepregnancy body mass index, weight gain during pregnancy, and perinatal outcome in a rural black population. J Matern Fetal Med 1998;7:190–193.
54 Wataba K, Mizutani T, Wasada K, Morine M, Sugiyama T, Suehara N: Impact of prepregnant body mass index and maternal weight gain on the risk of pregnancy complications in Japanese women. Acta Obstet Gynecol Scand 2006;85:269–276.
55 Ohlin A, Rossner S: Maternal body weight development after pregnancy. Int J Obes 1990;14:159–173.
56 Boardley DJ, Sargent RG, Coker AL, Hussey JR, Sharpe PA: The relationship between diet, activity, and other factors, and postpartum weight change by race. Obstet Gynecol 1995;86:834–838.
57 Schauberger CW, Rooney BL, Brimer LM: Factors that influence weight loss in the puerperium. Obstet Gynecol 1992;79:424–429.
58 Kac G, Benicio MH, Velasquez-Melendez G, Valente JG, Struchiner CJ: Gestational weight gain and prepregnancy weight influence postpartum weight retention in a cohort of Brazilian women. J Nutr 2004;134:661–666.
59 Keppel KG, Taffel SM: Pregnancy-related weight gain and retention: implications of the 1990 Institute of Medicine guidelines. Am J Public Health 1993;83:1100–1103.
60 Kleinman KP, Oken E, Radesky JS, Rich-Edwards JW, Peterson KE, Gillman MW: How should gestational weight gain be assessed? A comparison of existing methods and a novel method, area under the weight gain curve. Int J Epidemiol 2007;36:1275–1282.
61 Parker JD, Abrams B: Differences in postpartum weight retention between black and white mothers. Obstet Gynecol 1993;81:768–774.
62 Gunderson EP: Childbearing and obesity in women: weight before, during, and after pregnancy. Obstet Gynecol Clin North Am 2009;36:317–332.
63 Linne Y, Dye L, Barkeling B, Rossner S: Long-term weight development in women: A 15-year follow-up of the effects of pregnancy. Obes Res 2004;12:1166–1178.
64 Gunderson EP, Murtaugh MA, Lewis CE, Quesenberry CP, West DS, Sidney S: Excess gains in weight and waist circumference associated with childbearing: The Coronary Artery Risk Development in Young Adults Study (CARDIA). Int J Obes Relat Metab Disord 2004;28:525–535.

65 Gunderson EP, Lewis CE, Murtaugh MA, Quesenberry CP, Smith West D, Sidney S: Long-term plasma lipid changes associated with a first birth: The Coronary Artery Risk Development in Young Adults Study. Am J Epidemiol 2004;159:1028–1039.
66 Gunderson EP, Jacobs DR Jr, Chiang V, Lewis CE, Tsai A, Quesenberry CP Jr, Sidney S: Childbearing is associated with higher incidence of the metabolic syndrome among women of reproductive age controlling for measurements before pregnancy: the CARDIA study. Am J Obstet Gynecol 2009;201: 177.e1–177.e9.
67 Gunderson EP, Sternfeld B, Wellons MF, Whitmer RA, Chiang V, Quesenberry CP Jr, Lewis CE, Sidney S: Childbearing may increase visceral adipose tissue independent of overall increase in body fat. Obesity 2008;16: 1078–1084.
68 Weidner MD, Gavigan KE, Tyndall GL, Hickey MS, McCammon MR, Houmard JA: Which anthropometric indices of regional adiposity are related to the insulin resistance of aging? Int J Obes Relat Metab Disord 1995; 19:325–330.
69 Institute of Medicine: Nutrition During Pregnancy. Washington, National Academy Press, 1990.
70 Siega-Riz AM, Viswanathan M, Moos MK, Deierlein A, Mumford S, Knaack J, Thieda P, Lux LJ, Lohr KN: A systematic review of outcomes of maternal weight gain according to the Institute of Medicine recommendations: birth weight, fetal growth, and postpartum weight retention. Am J Obstet Gynecol 2009; 201:339.e1–339.e14.
71 Brown JE, Murtaugh MA, Jacobs DR Jr, Margellos HC: Variation in newborn size according to pregnancy weight change by trimester. Am J Clin Nutr 2002;76:205–209.
72 Neufeld LM, Haas JD, Grajeda R, Martorell R: Changes in maternal weight from the first to second trimester of pregnancy are associated with fetal growth and infant length at birth. Am J Clin Nutr 2004;79:646–652.
73 Catalano PM, Drago NM, Amini SB: Maternal carbohydrate metabolism and its relationship to fetal growth and body composition. Am J Obstet Gynecol 1995;172: 1464–1470.
74 Oken E, Kleinman KP, Belfort MB, Hammitt JK, Gillman MW: Associations of gestational weight gain with short- and longer-term maternal and child health outcomes. Am J Epidemiol 2009;170:173–180.
75 Hickey CA, McNeal SF, Menefee L, Ivey S: Prenatal weight gain within upper and lower recommended ranges: effect on birth weight of black and white infants. Obstet Gynecol 1997;90:489–494.
76 Sanin Aguirre LH, Reza-Lopez S, Levario-Carrillo M: Relation between maternal body composition and birth weight. Biol Neonate 2004;86:55–62.
77 Hutcheon JA, Platt RW, Meltzer SJ, Egeland GM: Is birth weight modified during pregnancy? Using sibling differences to understand the impact of blood glucose, obesity, and maternal weight gain in gestational diabetes. Am J Obstet Gynecol 2006;195:488–494.
78 Ananth CV, Wen SW: Trends in fetal growth among singleton gestations in the United States and Canada, 1985 through 1998. Semin Perinatol 2002;26:260–267.
79 Wen SW, Kramer MS, Platt R, Demissie K, Joseph KS, Liu S, Sauve R: Secular trends of fetal growth in Canada, 1981 to 1997. Paediatr Perinat Epidemiol 2003;17:347–354.
80 Kramer MS, Morin I, Yang H, Platt RW, Usher R, McNamara H, Joseph KS, Wen SW: Why are babies getting bigger? Temporal trends in fetal growth and its determinants. J Pediatr 2002;141:538–542.
81 Moreira P, Padez C, Mourao-Carvalhal I, Rosado V: Maternal weight gain during pregnancy and overweight in Portuguese children. Int J Obes (Lond) 2007;31:608–614.
82 Oken E, Rifas-Shiman SL, Field AE, Frazier AL, Gillman MW: Maternal gestational weight gain and offspring weight in adolescence. Obstet Gynecol 2008;112:999–1006.
83 Stuebe AM, Forman MR, Michels KB: Maternal-recalled gestational weight gain, prepregnancy body mass index, and obesity in the daughter. Int J Obes (Lond) 2009;33:743–752.
84 Schack-Nielsen L, Mortensen EL, Michaelsen KF, Sorensen TIA: High maternal pregnancy weight gain is associated with an increased risk of obesity in childhood and adulthood independent of maternal BMI (abstract). Pediatr Res 2005;58:1020.
85 Li C, Goran MI, Kaur H, Nollen N, Ahluwalia JS: Developmental trajectories of overweight during childhood: role of early life factors. Obesity (Silver Spring) 2007;15:760–771.
86 Whitaker RC: Predicting preschooler obesity at birth: the role of maternal obesity in early pregnancy. Pediatrics 2004;114:e29–e36.
87 Maffeis C, Micciolo R, Must A, Zaffanello M, Pinelli L: Parental and perinatal factors associated with childhood obesity in northeast Italy. Int J Obes Relat Metab Disord 1994;18:301–305.
88 Sharma AJ, Cogswell ME, Grummer-Strawn LM: The association between pregnancy weight gain is associated with an increased risk of obesity in childhood and adulthood independent of maternal BMI (abstract). Pediatr Res 2005;58:1038.
89 Kleiser C, Schaffrath Rosario A, Mensink GB, Prinz-Langenohl R, Kurth BM: Potential determinants of obesity among children and adolescents in Germany: results from the cross-sectional KIGGS study. BMC Public Health 2009;9:46.
90 McMillen IC, Edwards LJ, Duffield J, Muhlhausler BS: Regulation of leptin synthesis and secretion before birth: implications for the early programming of adult obesity. Reproduction 2006;131:415–427.
91 Shankar K, Harrell A, Liu X, Gilchrist JM, Ronis MJ, Badger TM: Maternal obesity at conception programs obesity in the offspring. Am J Physiol Regul Integr Comp Physiol 2008;294:R528–R538.
92 Samuelsson AM, Matthews PA, Argenton M, Christie MR, McConnell JM, Jansen EH, Piersma AH, Ozanne SE, Twinn DF, Remacle C, Rowlerson A, Poston L, Taylor PD: Diet-induced obesity in female mice leads to offspring hyperphagia, adiposity, hypertension, and insulin resistance: a novel murine model of developmental programming. Hypertension 2008;51:383–392.
93 Bayol SA, Farrington SJ, Stickland NC: A maternal 'junk food' diet in pregnancy and lactation promotes an exacerbated taste for 'junk food' and a greater propensity for obesity in rat offspring. Br J Nutr 2007;98: 843–851.
94 Wardle J, Guthrie C, Sanderson S, Birch L, Plomin R: Food and activity preferences in children of lean and obese parents. Int J Obes Relat Metab Disord 2001;25:971–977.
95 Rising R, Lifshitz F: Lower energy expenditures in infants from obese biological mothers. Nutr J 2008;7:15.
96 Muhlhausler BS, Duffield JA, McMillen IC: Increased maternal nutrition stimulates peroxisome proliferator activated receptor-γ, adiponectin, and leptin messenger ribonucleic acid expression in adipose tissue before birth. Endocrinology 2007;148: 878–885.
97 Muhlhausler BS, Adam CL, Findlay PA, Duffield JA, McMillen IC: Increased maternal nutrition alters development of the appetite-regulating network in the brain. FASEB J 2006;20:1257–1259.
98 Muhlhausler BS, Duffield JA, McMillen IC: Increased maternal nutrition increases leptin expression in perirenal and subcutaneous adipose tissue in the postnatal lamb. Endocrinology 2007;148:6157–6163.
99 Catalano PM: Obesity and pregnancy – the propagation of a viscous cycle? J Clin Endocrinol Metab 2003;88:3505–3506.
100 Spalding KL, Arner E, Westermark PO, Bernard S, Buchholz BA, Bergmann O, Blomqvist L, Hoffstedt J, Naslund E, Britton T, Concha H, Hassan M, Ryden M, Frisen J, Arner P: Dynamics of fat cell turnover in humans. Nature 2008;453:783–787.
101 Aagaard-Tillery KM, Grove K, Bishop J, Ke X, Fu Q, McKnight R, Lane RH: Developmental origins of disease and determinants of chromatin structure: maternal diet modifies the primate fetal epigenome. J Mol Endocrinol 2008;41:91–102.

102 Wu Q, Suzuki M: Parental obesity and overweight affect the body-fat accumulation in the offspring: the possible effect of a high-fat diet through epigenetic inheritance. Obes Rev 2006;7:201–208.
103 Bayol SA, Simbi BH, Stickland NC: A maternal cafeteria diet during gestation and lactation promotes adiposity and impairs skeletal muscle development and metabolism in rat offspring at weaning. J Physiol 2005;567:951–961.
104 Oken E, Guthrie L, Rifas-Shiman SL, Gillman MW: Maternal gestational weight gain and child cognition. Obesity (Silver Spring) 2009;17:S64.
105 Cogswell ME, Scanlon KS, Fein SB, Schieve LA: Medically advised, mother's personal target, and actual weight gain during pregnancy. Obstet Gynecol 1999;94:616–622.
106 Stotland NE, Haas JS, Brawarsky P, Jackson RA, Fuentes-Afflick E, Escobar GJ: Body mass index, provider advice, and target gestational weight gain. Obstet Gynecol 2005;105:633–638.
107 Asbee SM, Jenkins TR, Butler JR, White J, Elliot M, Rutledge A: Preventing excessive weight gain during pregnancy through dietary and lifestyle counseling: a randomized controlled trial. Obstet Gynecol 2009;113:305–312.
108 Olson CM, Strawderman MS, Reed RG: Efficacy of an intervention to prevent excessive gestational weight gain. Am J Obstet Gynecol 2004;191:530–536.
109 Kinnunen TI, Pasanen M, Aittasalo M, Fogelholm M, Weiderpass E, Luoto R: Reducing postpartum weight retention – a pilot trial in primary health care. Nutr J 2007;6:21.
110 Jeffries K, Shub A, Walker SP, Hiscock R, Permezel M: Reducing excessive weight gain in pregnancy: a randomised controlled trial. Med J Aust 2009;191:429–433.
111 Power ML, Cogswell ME, Schulkin J: Obesity prevention and treatment practices of US obstetrician-gynecologists. Obstet Gynecol 2006;108:961–968.
112 Herring SJ, Platek D, Elliott P, Riley L, Stuebe AM, Oken E: Addressing obesity in pregnancy: what do obstetric providers recommend? J Womens Health 2010;19:65–70.
113 Claesson IM, Sydsjo G, Brynhildsen J, Cedergren M, Jeppsson A, Nystrom F, Sydsjo A, Josefsson A: Weight gain restriction for obese pregnant women: a case-control intervention study. BJOG 2008;115:44–50.
114 Polley BA, Wing RR, Sims CJ: Randomized controlled trial to prevent excessive weight gain in pregnant women. Int J Obes Relat Metab Disord 2002;26:1494–1502.
115 Orstead C, Arrington D, Kamath SK, Olson R, Kohrs MB: Efficacy of prenatal nutrition counseling: weight gain, infant birth weight, and cost-effectiveness. J Am Diet Assoc 1985;85:40–45.

Annales Nestlé

Ann Nestlé [Engl] 2010;68:29–40
DOI: 10.1159/000298781

A Review of the Benefits of Nutrient Supplements during Pregnancy: From Iron-Folic-Acid to Long-Chain Polyunsaturated Fatty Acids to Probiotics

Usha Ramakrishnan

Hubert Department of Global Health, Rollins School of Public Health, Emory University, Atlanta, Ga., USA

Key Words
Nutrient supplements, pregnancy · Iron-folic-acid · Probiotics

Abstract
This review summarizes current knowledge on the effectiveness of prenatal nutrient supplements ranging from iron-folic-acid (IFA), which is standard of care in many parts of the world, to more novel ones such as ω–3 fatty acids and probiotics in improving maternal and child health outcomes. Randomized controlled trials have shown that prenatal IFA supplements reduce the risk of anemia and iron deficiency during pregnancy and at term, but the evidence of risk reductions in low birth weight (LBW) and preterm delivery (PTD) is weak. Recent studies, however, suggest that prenatal IFA supplements may reduce child mortality. On the other hand, there is convincing evidence that multiple micronutrient supplements containing 1–2 recommended daily allowances of several vitamins and minerals are safe and reduce the risk of LBW by 19 and 17% when compared to a placebo or routine IFA. Prenatal calcium supplements (>1 g/day) have also been shown to significantly reduce the risk of preeclampsia and maternal death or serious morbidity by 52 and 20%, respectively. Zinc and fish oil supplements containing ω–3 fatty acids may also increase gestational age and reduce the risk of PTD, but not of LBW, in selected populations. There is, however, limited evidence to support the provision of supplements containing only vitamin A, D or antioxidants such as vitamins C and E. Although the protective effect of folic acid during the periconceptual period in reducing neural tube defects is well established, very few or no intervention trials have evaluated the independent effects of specific B vitamins (vitamins B_6, B_{12} and folic acid), docosahexanoic acid and probiotics during pregnancy. The effects of prenatal iodine supplements in areas with mild to moderate iodine deficiency have not been examined either. Some of these nutrients may not affect outcomes such as PTD or LBW but may have long-term benefits for offspring health and development.

Introduction

Adverse pregnancy outcomes such as maternal mortality, preterm delivery (PTD) and intrauterine growth retardation remain significant public health problems especially in resource-poor environments where access to quality care and food are limited [1]. Low birth weight

KARGER

Fax +41 61 306 12 34
E-Mail karger@karger.ch
www.karger.com

0517–8606/10/0681–0029$26.00/0

Accessible online at:
www.karger.com/ane

Usha Ramakrishnan, PhD, Associate Professor
Hubert Department of Global Health
Rollins School of Public Health, Emory University
Atlanta GA 30322 (USA)
Tel. +1 404 727 1092, Fax +1 404 727 1278, E-Mail uramakr@emory.edu

Table 1. Effect of nutrient interventions during pregnancy on maternal and child health outcomes [3]

Sufficient evidence for implementation	Interventions with insufficient or variable evidence of effectiveness	Interventions for which evidence showed no or little effect
Iron-folate	Iodine	Zinc
Multiple micronutrient	Vitamin A	Vitamin D
Calcium		Pyridoxine
		Fish oil

(LBW, i.e. <2.5 kg) affects ~13 million births each year and is associated with a range of both short- and long-term consequences such as increased morbidity and mortality and decreased intellectual potential [2]. Considerable attention has been paid to the importance of nutrition during pregnancy in both developed and developing countries. More recently, several intervention trials have evaluated the benefits of providing nutrient supplements that range from single nutrients such as vitamin A to combinations such as multivitamin-mineral supplements and fish oil supplements that are a rich source of ω–3 fatty acids. In a recent global review of interventions that affect maternal and child undernutrition and survival, Bhutta et al. [3] concluded that there was sufficient evidence of the benefit of the provision of iron-folate (IFA), multiple micronutrient (MMN) and calcium supplements to pregnant women in the 36 countries that account for the majority of undernourished children. They also identified nutrient interventions with variable or no evidence of benefit as shown in table 1.

This review is an update of the literature and focuses on the evidence of the benefits of prenatal nutrient supplements on a wider range of maternal and child health outcomes that are of concern in both developed and developing countries. For example, the evidence on the benefits of antioxidants and probiotics has been included. The implications of prenatal interventions for outcomes such as postnatal growth and development and the development of chronic conditions such as allergy and asthma have also been addressed. Although studies have examined the benefits of improving nutrient intakes either by the provision of food-based supplements that provide additional energy as well as macronutrients like fat and protein and several micronutrients, and/or by nutrition education, these interventions have not been included in this review.

Iron and Folic Acid

Iron is one of the nutrients whose requirements increase dramatically during pregnancy due to increased blood volume expansion and new tissues. Approximately 6 mg/day is needed during gestation compared to only 1.3 mg/day among nonpregnant women of reproductive age (WRA). Although iron absorption is increased, concerns have been expressed about the ability of diet alone to meet this greater demand especially in settings where iron deficiency is common in women even before they get pregnant [4]. Current recommendations for prenatal iron supplementation exist even in developed countries, where the prevalences of anemia and iron deficiency are much lower than in developing countries. For example, all women are recommended to consume a daily supplement containing 30 mg of iron during the last trimester of pregnancy in the USA and selective supplementation with higher doses may be provided earlier for women who are diagnosed as anemic or iron deficient [5]. The World Health Organization (WHO) has a universal recommendation for all pregnant women to consume a daily supplement that contains 60 mg of iron and 400 μg of folic acid, which is important for many developing countries, where anemia and iron deficiency are common [6]. In addition to the direct effects of anemia, such as fatigue and reduced work capacity, iron deficiency and anemia during pregnancy have been associated with poor birth outcomes including small for gestational age (SGA) and PTD. Most of the evidence, however, has been based on observational studies and not corroborated by findings from well-designed placebo-controlled randomized controlled trials (RCTs) [4]. In a recent systematic review, Peña-Rosas and Viteri [7] carefully evaluated the existing evidence (as of June 2009) on whether routine intake of supplements containing iron or a combination of iron and folic acid during pregnancy improves a wide range of maternal health and pregnancy outcomes. This review included a total of 49 trials (randomized and quasi-randomized) involving 23,200 pregnant women and the key conclusions were as follows.

- Women who received daily prenatal iron supplementation with or without folic acid were less likely to have iron deficiency and anemia during pregnancy and at term compared to those who received a placebo or no treatment.
- Side effects and hemoconcentration are more common in women who receive daily iron supplementation.

- There were no differences in the effects of daily and weekly supplementation on gestational anemia.
- There is no evidence of significant reduction in maternal and neonatal outcomes such as LBW, preterm birth, infection, delayed development and postpartum hemorrhage.

These findings, which are similar to an earlier review by the same authors, have led to the consideration of weekly supplementation during pregnancy as an alternate and safer approach to current practice of daily supplementation. The implications of increased hemoconcentration seen among women who consumed IFA daily are unclear, but there are practical advantages to promoting using weekly supplements in terms of reduced costs and perhaps increased compliance, which in turn may increase the cost-effectiveness. Although current recommendations for pregnant women are unlikely to change, the WHO recently made a recommendation for the provision of weekly IFA supplements to all WRA in areas where iron deficiency and anemia are significant public health problems [8]. Despite the paucity of data on the long-term benefits for maternal and child health outcomes, the expectation is that this approach would help improve the preconceptual nutritional status, which in turn would result in improved pregnancy outcomes.

It should also be noted that while the last conclusion does not support the recommendations made by Bhutta et al. [1], data on the impact of daily prenatal IFA on maternal and neonatal outcomes such as LBW are limited and there is considerable heterogeneity across studies. Only 9 (n = 6,275) out of the 49 trials included in the systematic review had data on birth size and showed a 21% reduction in the risk of LBW for those who received daily iron supplements compared to those who received no iron or placebo that was not statistically significant [risk ratio (RR) = 0.79; 95% confidence interval (CI) = 0.61–1.03]. The same was true for PTD that was based on 8 trials (n = 5,730); a 15% reduction in risk of PTD was seen among the iron-treated groups compared to placebo or no treatment, but it was not statistically significant (RR = 0.85; 95% CI = 0.67–1.09). Even fewer studies have examined maternal outcomes such as preeclampsia or mortality, indicating the need for well-designed large trials. Interestingly, the authors report that their findings for birth weight did not change when they restricted the analysis to the high-quality studies (n = 7), but it was statistically significant (RR = 0.82, 95% CI = 0.71–0.94) when the analysis was restricted to the 3 trials (n = 1,823) that had unspecified or mixed anemic status. They also found significant differences for birth length [weighted mean difference (WMD) = 0.38 cm, 95% CI = 0.10–0.65 cm], which was reported in 5 out of the 9 studies included in the birth weight analysis. The authors call for more research and the findings of several large ongoing RCTs will play an important role in confirming the effect of prenatal IFA on reducing the burden of LBW and PTD. The findings of one of these studies that was not included in the meta-analysis are described here [9]. A large double-blind RCT was conducted in rural North-West China in which villages were randomized for all pregnant women to take either daily folic acid (control), IFA or MMN with a recommended allowance of 15 vitamins and minerals. Relative to folic acid alone, prenatal IFA supplementation was associated with a 50% reduction in the risk of early PTD (<34 weeks) (RR = 0.50, 95% CI = 0.27–0.94) and a 54% reduction in the risk of early neonatal mortality (RR = 0.46, 95% CI = 0.21–0.98). There was no significant effect on LBW (RR = 0.81, 95% CI = 0.59–1.12), which was 4.5 and 5.3% in the IFA and folic-acid groups. The birth length, however, was significantly greater in the IFA group compared to the folic acid group (WMD = 0.24 cm, 95% CI = 0.02–0.46 cm). Long-term benefits of prenatal IFA supplementation have also been reported in a recent follow-up of a large cluster randomized trial in Nepal in which the efficacy of 4 different combinations of antenatal micronutrient supplements, namely folic acid only, IFA, IFA-zinc and a multivitamin-mineral supplement were compared [10]. The percentage of LBW infants was significantly lower in the group that received IFA supplements (34%) compared to the control group (43%) that received only vitamin A (RR = 0.84, 95% CI = 0.72–0.99]. Although there were no differences in the prevalence of PTD or neonatal morbidity in the first 10 days of life or at 6 weeks of age [11], the offspring of women who received IFA supplements during pregnancy were less likely to die in the first 7 years of of life [hazard ratio (HR) = 0.69; 95% CI = 0.49–0.99] compared to those who received a placebo [12]. These reductions in child mortality in 2 varied settings provide valuable data for improving ongoing efforts to augment antenatal care and consumption of prenatal IFA supplements. The strengths of both these studies include the large sample size, the range of outcomes examined and low loss to follow-up.

Finally, the importance of just folic acid during the periconceptual period in the prevention of neural tube defects (NTDs) is well recognized and has led to worldwide efforts to improve folic acid intakes in WRA [13]. Mandatory fortification of flour with folic acid in coun-

Table 2. Description of trials that examined the benefits of prenatal multivitamin-mineral supplements

Study site	Study period	Sample description	Experimental groups	Control group	Weeks pregnant at recruitment
Tanzania [20]	1995–1997	257–270 per group HIV+ women	1. MMN with vitamin A (+ 9 other nutrients) 2. MMN without vitamin A (+ 9 other nutrients) 3. Vitamin A only 120 mg Fe + 5 mg FA also given to all groups	Placebo 120 mg Fe + 5 mg FA also given	25–32
Zimbabwe [21]	1996–1997	832–837 per group	MMN with 13 nutrients	Placebo Fe FA offered as part of antenatal care	25–32
Mexico [16]	1997–2000	322–323 per group	MMN with 13 nutrients	60 mg Fe	<13
Sarlahi, Nepal [10, 11]	1998–2001	772–876 per group	1. Vitamin A + FA 2. MMN with vitamin A + FA + Fe 3. MMN with vitamin A + FA + Fe + Zn 4. MMN with 15 nutrients	1,000 μg RE vitamin A	9–17
France [22]	2001	32–33 per group	MMN with 12 nutrients	Placebo	12–16
Guinea-Bissau [23]	2001–2002	519–542 per group	1. MMN with 13 nutrients 2. Two MMN daily	60 mg Fe + 400 μg FA	<37
Indonesia [18]	2001–2004	2,543–21,296 per group	MMN (UNIMMAP)[1]	30 mg Fe and 400 μg FA	At any gestational age
Tanzania [24]	2001–2004	4,000 per group HIV– women	Multivitamin (no vitamin A; 2–10 RDA)	Placebo, all received 60 mg Fe and 250 μg FA	12–27
India [25]	2002–2003	99–101 per group	MMN (with 29 vitamins and minerals)	Placebo (+ 60 mg Fe and 500 μg FA)	24–32
Janakpur, (Central) Nepal [26]	2002–2004	517–537 per group	MMN with 13 nutrients	60 mg Fe + 400 μg FA	≤20
China [9]	2002–2006	1,899–2,017 per group	MMN[1], 60 mg Fe + 400 μg FA	400 μg FA only	<28
Niger [19]	2004–2005	1,777–1,893 per group	MMN (UNIMMAP)[1]	60 mg Fe and 400 μg FA	<12
Rural Burkina Faso [17]	2004–2006	712–714 per group	MMN (UNIMMAP)[1]	30 mg Fe and 400 μg FA	At any gestational age[2]

FA = Folic acid; RE = retinol equivalent; RDA = recommended daily allowance.

[1] The UNIMMAP supplement contained 1 RDA of vitamin A, vitamin B_1, vitamin B_2, niacin, vitamin B_6, vitamin B_{12}, folic acid, vitamin C, vitamin D, vitamin E, copper, selenium, iodine; with 30 mg Fe and 15 mg zinc.

[2] One third of the women were in the first trimester, half were in the second trimester, and the remainder were in the third trimester.

tries such as the USA have resulted in significant reductions in birth defects, especially NTDs [14]. However, much less is known about the importance of folic acid later in gestation. Folic acid results in megaloblastic anemia and may be associated with birth size. Christian et al. [10] found no effects of folic acid only on birth size but did find a reduced risk of mortality from birth to 7 years in the folic acid-only group compared to the placebo.

Multiple Micronutrients

Deficiencies of MMN usually coexist in many developing countries, which led to considerable interest by researchers and implementors in evaluating the benefits of providing pregnant women with a daily MMN supplement that contains several vitamins and minerals. In an earlier meta-analysis that included 9 trials (n = 15,378 women), Haider and Bhutta [15] reported that prenatal MMN supplementation reduced the risk of LBW by 17%

(RR = 0.83; 95% CI = 0.76–0.9) when they compared supplementation of 2 or less micronutrients to no supplementation or a placebo. Significant reductions were also seen for SGA births (RR = 0.92; 95% CI = 0.86–0.99) and anemia (RR = 0.61; 95% CI = 0.52–0.71). These effects, however, were not statistically significant when they compared MMN supplementation to IFA (RR for LBW = 0.94; 95% CI = 0.83–1.06; SGA RR = 1.04; 95% CI = 0.93–1.17). There were no differences for preterm births and perinatal mortality either. This review, however, did not include several recently completed studies.

A brief description of the controlled trials [9–11, 16–26] that have evaluated the effects of prenatal MMN supplements is provided in table 2. These studies were conducted primarily in developing countries with a wide range of baseline prevalence of LBW and only 1 study was conducted in a developed country, namely France [22]. Many of them compared a daily prenatal MMN supplement containing 1–2 times the recommended daily allowance for several vitamins (A, B complex, C, D and E) and trace elements such as iron, zinc and copper to the standard IFA supplement. Although some of the early studies [10, 16] did not find significant differences in birth size among women who received MMN supplements when compared to iron, recent studies have shown otherwise [17–19]. Of particular note is the large double-blind cluster-randomised trial that was conducted in Indonesia [18]. Midwives were advised to distribute either IFA or MMN supplements (UNIMMAP supplement) in a randomized fashion to pregnant women who consumed the supplements daily up to delivery and during the first 3 months postpartum. Intention to treat analysis revealed an 18% reduction (RR = 0.82, 95% CI = 0.70–0.95) in early infant mortality among infants born to women consuming MMN supplements compared to those who consumed IFA supplements. Combined fetal loss and neonatal deaths were also reduced by 11% (RR = 0.89, 95% CI = 0.81–1.00), with significant effects in undernourished (RR = 0.85, 95% CI = 0.73–0.98) or anemic (RR = 0.71, 95% CI = 0.58–0.87) women. This study also showed that the reductions in the risk of LBW were greatest among those infants born to women who were anemic at baseline; the overall reduction was 14% (RR = 0.86, 95% CI = 0.73–1.01) for those in the MMN group compared to the IFA group and 33% (RR = 0.67, 95% CI = 0.51–0.89) for infants of women who were anemic at enrolment. The other recent large trial was conducted in North West China [9]. This study did not find any significant differences in the risk of LBW (RR = 0.78, 95% CI = 0.56–1.08) or PTD (RR = 0.86, 95% CI = 0.64–1.14), but there were significant increases in mean birth weight and gestational age in the MMN group compared to the folic acid-only group. There were no significant differences in perinatal mortality (stillbirths and early neonatal mortality) between the 3 groups either. The findings of these 2 recent studies [9, 18] have assuaged earlier concerns that MMN supplementation may increase infant mortality [27] and confirm the benefits of providing pregnant women with MMN supplements especially in settings where anemia and undernutrition are common. In a more recent systematic review that included the results of all the 13 MMN trials published to date, Shah et al. [28] estimated a 19% reduction in the prevalence of LBW that could be attributed to prenatal MMN in comparison to a placebo (RR = 0.81, 95% CI = 0.73–0.91). More importantly, there was a significant reduction in the risk of LBW even when prenatal MMN supplementation was compared to IFA supplementation (RR = 0.83, 95% CI = 0.74–0.93) and birth weight was significantly higher (WMD = 54 g; 95% CI = 36–72 g) among infants whose mothers were in the MMN group compared to those in the IFA group. There were, however, no differences in PTD. In summary, the evidence clearly supports the implementation of a recommendation to provide MMN supplements to pregnant women especially in settings where LBW continues to be a significant public health problem.

Calcium

Hypertension is a major complication of pregnancy and several studies have evaluated the benefits of calcium supplementation in reducing the risk of pregnancy-related hypertension and associated complications. A recent meta-analysis [29] showed that prenatal Ca supplementation (≥1 g/day) significantly reduced the risk of high blood pressure by 30% (95% CI = 14–43), preeclampsia by 52% (95% CI = 31–67) and maternal death or serious morbidity by 20% (95% CI = 3–35) when compared to a placebo (12 trials; n = 15,528). There were, however, no significant differences in the risk for PTD and still births, which were reduced by 19 and 11%, respectively. One concern with the interpretation of these findings is possible publication bias. Prenatal Ca supplementation (1.5 g/day) did not significantly reduce the risk of preeclampsia (RR = 0.91, 95% CI = 0.69–1.19) in a large (n = 8,325) high-quality WHO multicenter trial that was conducted in developing country settings where calcium intakes were low [30] and included in the meta-analysis. There were, however, significant reductions in the risk of severe gestational hypertension (RR = 0.71; 95% CI = 0.61–0.82), eclampsia (RR = 0.68; 95% CI = 0.48–0.97) and neonatal mortality (RR = 0.70; 95% CI = 0.56–0.88). The risk for PTD was also significantly reduced among younger women (<20 years). A recent trial conducted in India [31] has also shown significant benefits of Ca supplementation in reducing the risks of preeclampsia, high blood pressure and even preterm births. This study used a higher dose (2 g/day) and was also done among nulliparous women with low intakes of dietary Ca (~300 mg/day) similar to the WHO trial. In summary, studies conducted to date are suggestive of benefits to maternal and child health outcomes especially in settings with low Ca intakes.

Magnesium

There is some evidence suggesting benefits of providing magnesium during pregnancy. In a meta-analysis that included 5 trials, Makrides and Crowther [32] estimated that compared to a placebo, oral magnesium supplements before 25 weeks gestation were associated with a 27% reduction in the rate of PTD (RR = 0.73; 95% CI = 0.57–0.94; n = 2,275). Similar reductions were seen for the rate of LBW (RR = 0.70; 95% CI = 0.53–0.93; n = 1,741). All the studies were conducted in developed countries (USA, Hungary and Austria) and the authors judged only 1 study to be of high quality, raising the possibility of biased results. Of note is the lack of significant differences in mean gestational age (WMD = 0.11, 95% CI = –0.06 to 0.29 days) or birth weight (WMD = 50.8, 95% CI = –0.2 to 101.9 g) and the effects on PTD and SGA were not significant following the exclusion of a large cluster randomized trial from Hungary (n = 985). These findings suggest that there is limited high-quality evidence regarding the benefits of oral magnesium supplements during pregnancy and the value of including magnesium in routine prenatal supplements remains to be evaluated.

Iodine

Severe iodine deficiency has long been associated with adverse pregnancy outcomes including pregnancy loss, still birth and irreversible brain damage that results in cretinism. Early studies conducted in areas where severe iodine deficiency is endemic have demonstrated the benefits of providing iodine during pregnancy, primarily as injectable or oral iodized oil, in reducing the rates of endemic cretinism [33]. In contrast, little work has been done on the benefits of providing iodine supplements in women with mild to moderate iodine deficiency. A few trials have shown that iodine supplementation was effective in minimizing an increase in thyroid size during pregnancy, but none have examined outcomes such as LBW or health and development of the offspring. The other concern is related to the safety of providing iodine supplements (either alone or as part of MMN supplement) in the context of universal salt iodization, which has been a successful strategy to eliminate iodine deficiency disorders. Current WHO recommendations for pregnant women living in settings where <90% are using iodized salt and the median urinary iodine in school age children <100 μg/l indicate a single annual dose of iodized oil containing 400 mg or a daily dose of 250 μg/I as potassium iodide. Pregnant women who have received iodized oil during their current pregnancy or up to 3 months before the current pregnancy should not consume iodine supplements [33].

Vitamin A

Vitamin A deficiency is common during pregnancy in many developing countries and although its role in child health is well known, concerns about the safety of providing vitamin A supplements during pregnancy remain [34]. Recent interest in the role of vitamin A in reducing the risk of mother-to-child transmission (MTCT) of HIV has led to several studies primarily in Subsaharan Africa. In a recent meta-analysis, however, Kongnyuy et al. [35] found no evidence of benefit of vitamin A on the risk of MTCT of HIV (RR = 1.06, 95% CI = 0.89–1.26; n = 7,528) based on the findings of 3 trials that provided oral vitamin A daily [36–38] during pregnancy and 1 trial in Zimbabwe that provided a large single dose of oral vitamin A for the mother (400,000 IU) and newborn (50,000 IU) soon after delivery [39]. The trials conducted in South Africa [36] and Malawi [38] did not find evidence of benefit, but the trial in Tanzania [37] showed that vitamin A supplementation increased the risk of MTCT of HIV by 53% (OR = 1.53, 95% CI = 1.15–2.04) by 24 months of age and raised concerns about the safety of prenatal vitamin A supplementation in HIV-infected women. There was no evidence of effects on other pregnancy outcomes either, namely stillbirths (RR = 0.99; 95% CI = 0.68–1.43), PTD (RR = 0.88; 95% CI = 0.65–1.19), death before 24 months among live births (RR = 1.08; 95% CI = 0.91–1.29) and maternal death (RR = 0.83; 95% CI = 0.59–1.17). Interestingly, the meta-analysis showed that prenatal vitamin A supplementation significantly improved birth weight (WMD = 89.78 g; 95% CI = 84.73–94.83 g). Villamor et al. [40], who followed up the offspring in the Tanzania study in which prenatal vitamins and not vitamin A improved birth size [20], found that children whose mothers received prenatal multivitamins were significantly heavier at 2 years of age (459 g; 95% CI = 35–882 g) and vitamin A seemed to reduce the benefits of multivitamins on these outcomes. Finally, very few studies have evaluated the benefits of prenatal vitamin A supplements on pregnancy outcomes in other parts of the world where the prevalence of HIV is much lower but vitamin A deficiency and LBW are high. A large cluster RCT that was conducted in Nepal found dramatic reductions in maternal mortality (~40%) among the women who received a weekly supplement of either vitamin A or β-carotene compared to placebo from early pregnancy through the first 6 weeks postpartum [41]. These findings, however, were not replicated in a similar large trial that was conducted in Bangladesh [34], and the effects on other outcomes such as PTD or LBW have not been published. In summary, the evidence to date does not support the large-scale distribution of prenatal vitamin A-only supplements even in settings where vitamin A deficiency is common. This does not, however, preclude the inclusion of this important vitamin in multivitamin supplements as it could help improve maternal and neonatal health.

Zinc

Zinc is an important micronutrient for normal growth and development and zinc deficiency during pregnancy has been associated with pregnancy loss and poor birth outcomes [42]. Several controlled trials of prenatal zinc supplementation have been conducted with mixed findings. In a systematic review that included 17 RCTs, Mahomed et al. [43] reported that prenatal Zn supplementation resulted in a 14% reduction in preterm birth (RR = 0.86; 95% CI = 0.76–0.98 in 13 RCTs; 6,854 women) and in a small effect favoring zinc for caesarean section (4 trials with high heterogeneity). There were, however, no significant differences in LBW (RR = 1.05; 95% Cl = 0.94–1.17; 11 studies of 4,941 women) or other maternal or neonatal outcomes. Although zinc supplementation during infancy has been shown to reduce child morbidity [3], the few trials that have examined maternal morbidity report mixed findings [42]. There is also some evidence that prenatal Zn supplementation may reduce infant morbidity and influence child growth and development even though the birth size is unaffected [42]. Finally, a recent case-control study found that high maternal serum levels of copper and low levels of zinc during pregnancy were positively associated with NTD in newborns [44], indicating the possible role of zinc during early pregnancy. In summary, although current findings suggest limited benefits for prenatal Zn supplementation, there may be subgroups who are likely to benefit and the recommendation made by Hess and King [42] for more research 'to assess the benefits of the large-scale introduction of zinc supplementation during pregnancy on congenital malformations, immune functions, neurobehavior, and overall neonatal survival in countries where zinc deficiency is a problem' is timely. The value of providing zinc in MMN supplements also needs to be evaluated in light of the potential interactions with other nutrients.

Vitamin D

Vitamin D is needed for the absorption and utilization of calcium, may influence fetal growth and can also influence immune function. Although there has been considerable interest in vitamin D in recent years, little is known about the value of providing vitamin D supplements during pregnancy besides being part of standard multivitamin-mineral supplements. No intervention trials evaluating the effects of prenatal supplements containing only vitamin D were identified. However, the findings of a well-designed prospective study suggest that maternal intake of vitamin D during pregnancy may be associated with preventing allergic diseases in the offspring [45]. Maternal vitamin D intakes during pregnancy were assessed using a food frequency questionnaire from food and supplements, and related to the prevalence of asthma, allergic rhinitis and atopic eczema by the age of 5 years in the offspring with HLA-DQB1-conferred susceptibility for type 1 diabetes. Maternal intake of vitamin D from food was negatively related to risk of asthma (HR = 0.80; 95% CI = 0.64–30.99) and allergic rhinitis (HR = 0.85; 95% CI = 0.75–30.97), but the consumption of vitamin D supplements alone was not associated with any outcome.

Antioxidants

There has been considerable interest in the benefits and risks of consuming supplements containing antioxidants, especially vitamins C and E, during pregnancy.

The key outcomes of interest concern preeclampsia and PTD. Preeclampsia is a serious complication of pregnancy which increases the risk of dying for both mother and infant and may lead to intrauterine growth retardation and premature birth. A possible contributing factor to the development of preeclampsia may be the presence of excessive amounts of chemicals called 'free radicals', which is why antioxidants, such as vitamin C, vitamin E, selenium and lycopene, may be protective as they can neutralize free radicals. PTD may also result from rupture of membranes and/or infections which may be affected by antioxidants. Based on a systematic review that included 10 RCTs (n = 6,533), Rumbold et al. [46] concluded that antioxidants during pregnancy did not reduce the risk of preeclampsia (RR = 0.73, 95% CI = 0.51–1.06) or other complications in pregnancy. The studies used varying combinations of antioxidants that were primarily vitamins; 1 study used the mineral selenium. Few trials, however, examined birth outcomes such as PTD and SGA. When antioxidants were assessed separately, there were insufficient data to be clear about whether there was any benefit or not, except for vitamins C and E. It should be noted, however, that several studies were still underway when this meta-analysis was conducted and some of the findings have been published since. Of particular interest is the recent WHO multicenter randomized trial of supplementation with vitamins C and E among pregnant women at high risk for preeclampsia in populations of low nutritional status from developing countries [47]. Pregnant women were randomized to receive 1,000 mg of vitamin C along with 400 IU of vitamin E or a placebo from 14 to 26 weeks' gestation up to delivery and followed up for birth outcomes. The study sites included Trujillo, Peru, Nagpur, India, Cape Town, South Africa and Ho Chi Minh City, Vietnam. A total of 1,265 women were randomized to treatment; loss to follow-up was low (<2%) and compliance was 87%. No differences were seen in preeclampsia (RR = 1.0; 95% CI = 0.9–1.3), eclampsia (RR = 1.5; 95% CI = 0.3–8.9), gestational hypertension (RR = 1.2; 95% CI = 0.9–1.7) nor any other maternal outcome. Rates of LBW (RR = 0.9; 95% CI = 0.8–1.1), SGA (RR = 0.9; 95% CI = 0.8–1.1) and perinatal deaths (RR = 0.8; 95% CI = 0.6–1.2) were also unaffected. These findings clearly support the earlier conclusion that antioxidants, especially vitamins C and E, do not provide any benefits for maternal and birth outcomes.

Long-Chain Polyunsaturated Fatty Acids

There has been considerable interest in the importance of long-chain polyunsaturated fatty acids (LCPUFAs), especially the ω–3 fatty acids for fetal development. Docosahexanoic acid (DHA) in particular is an important ω–3 fatty acid which accumulates rapidly in the brain and retina during gestation and the first year of life and is an important component of neural and retinal membranes [48]. Although humans can synthesize DHA from the parent 18 carbon ω–3 fatty acid, α-linoleic acid, there have been concerns about the efficiency of this process and possible competition with ω–6 fatty acids for the same enzymes. This has led to recommendations to ensure adequate consumption of preformed DHA in the diet, especially for pregnant women and young children. Based on a review of the literature that evaluated current knowledge on the role of LCPUFAs, especially DHA in maternal and infant nutrition, it was agreed that pregnant and lactating women should aim to achieve an average daily intake of at least 200 mg of DHA [49]. These recommendations were based primarily on the findings of recent meta-analyses [50, 51] that demonstrated that the consumption of fish oils rich in ω–3 LCPUFA during pregnancy reduces the risk for early premature birth. Szajewska et al. [51] identified 6 RCTs (n = 1,278) that compared the effects of prenatal LCPUFA supplementation with a placebo or no supplementation on pregnancy outcomes and size at birth and found that LCPUFA supplementation significantly increased the duration of pregnancy by 1.57 days (95% CI = 0.35–2.78) compared to controls among low-risk pregnancies. Interestingly, only 1 study was at low risk of bias and there was no evidence that supplementation reduced the risk of preeclampsia, PTD or LBW infants. There was a significant increase in head circumference, but the effect was small (WMD = 0.26 cm; 95% CI = 0.02–0.49 cm; n = 729) and disappeared in the sensitivity analysis. There were no significant differences in birth weight (WMD = 54 g; 95% CI = –3.1 to 111 g) in 5 RCTs (1,262 infants) and in birth length (WMD = 0.23 cm; 95% CI = –0.04 to 0.5 cm). A few trials have, however, been completed since this meta-analysis. The benefits of providing daily supplements containing fish oil (0.5 g of DHA and 0.15 g of eicosapentaenoic acid) and methyltetrahydrofolic acid (400 μg) from midgestation up to delivery was evaluated in a recent multicenter study (n = 311) in 3 European countries (Germany, Hungary and Spain). There were no differences in pregnancy outcomes and fetal development, even though fish oil significantly ($p < 0.001$) increased cord blood DHA and methyltetrahydrofolic acid was significantly associated ($p < 0.05$) with increased maternal DHA (percent by weight) [52]. A key limitation is the inadequate sample size to detect significant differences in birth outcomes such as gestational age and birth weight. A recently completed large trial (n = 1,094) also failed to detect any differences in gestational age or birth size among the offspring of women who received 400 mg of algal DHA compared to placebo from midpregnancy up to delivery. There was, however, a suggestion of benefit in birth weight and head circumference in the offspring of primiparous women who received DHA compared to placebo [53]. In another meta-analysis that focused on high-risk pregnancies [50], prenatal LCPUFA supplementation did not affect the duration of gestation, birth weight or other adverse pregnancy outcomes such as pregnancy-induced hypertension or preeclampsia, but was associated with a 61% reduction (RR = 0.39; 95% CI = 0.18–0.84) in the risk of early PTD (<34 weeks); this estimate was, however, based only on 2 RCTs (n = 391). Another limitation is the heterogeneity in the treatment that varied from study to study.

Observational studies and a few intervention trials suggest that higher maternal DHA intake both in pregnancy and lactation is associated with positive infant neurodevelopmental outcomes [48]. In a large prospective study, Hibbeln et al. [54] showed that low or no maternal seafood intake during pregnancy was a risk factor for lower verbal IQ (at 8 years) and suboptimal prosocial behavior (at 7 years), fine motor skills (at 18 and 42 months), communication (at 6 and 18 months) and social development (at 30 and 42 months) scores in the offspring. More importantly, follow-up of infants born to women who participated in an RCT in Norway showed that offspring of women who received the fish oil supplements from midgestation and through the first 3 months postpartum had improved scores in mental processing tests carried out at 4 years of age compared to those born to women who received the placebo. Loss to follow-up was, however, high [55]. Another follow-up of children born to atopic Australian women who participated in an RCT also showed that children of the fish-oil-supplemented mothers achieved significantly higher scores on the eye and hand coordination test compared to the control group at 2.5 years of age [56]. In summary, very few studies have evaluated the benefits of providing only DHA and the role of the balance of fatty acid intake, i.e., ω–3:ω–6 ratio. Little is also known on the benefits of prenatal LCPUFA supplementation on subsequent infant outcomes, although a few studies suggest that changes in maternal intake of ω–3 PUFAs, especially DHA, during pregnancy are positively associated with cognitive performance later on.

Probiotics

There has been considerable interest in the benefits of probiotics, especially in the prevention of atopic disease and allergy in young children. In a recent review, however, Kopp et al. [57] concluded that there was insufficient evidence to recommend probiotics during pregnancy and early infancy for the prevention of atopic disease and that more research was needed to identify subgroups that may benefit from the use of selected probiotic strains. A major limitation of the studies conducted to date is the variation in the treatment and study design. Probiotics also include a wide range of different bacteriological strains and species and vary in their protective abilities. Studies also differ in the outcomes measured and the timing of the intervention which begins during pregnancy and may continue during lactation in the mother and/or neonate. Furthermore, the few studies with comparable designs have different findings. Kalliomaki et al. [58] reported a 50% reduction in the frequency of atopic dermatitis among neonates treated with *Lactobacillus rhamnosus* GG in a randomized placebo-controlled trial that followed up the children till 7 years of age, whereas Kopp et al. [57] failed to confirm these findings. Nevertheless, studies conducted to date are suggestive of benefits especially in the immunomodulatory effects in neonates. Probiotics during pregnancy may influence the composition of breastmilk and reduce the incidence of IgE-associated eczema in infancy [59]. Since probiotics have anti-infective properties, they may also play a role in preventing PTD by killing pathogens and interrupting the role of inflammation and infection in preterm labor and delivery. Several probiotic preparations containing selected strains of lactobacilli are commercially available for treating bacterial vaginosis, yeast infections and urinary tract infections in WRA and are currently recommended for the treatment of bacterial vaginosis in high-risk pregnant women. These preparations may be administered either vaginally or orally and have been shown to be effective in reducing urogenital infections. In a recent meta-analysis, Othman et al. [60] reported an 81% reduction in the risk of genital infections (RR = 0.19; 95% CI = 0.08–0.48) when probiotics were used during pregnancy (oral or local treatment), but data on PTD and complications are lacking. Only 2 trials, however, were included in their systematic review; one enrolled women after 34 weeks of pregnancy using oral fermented milk as probiotic, while the other study utilized commercially available yogurt to be used vaginally by women diagnosed as having bacterial vaginosis in early pregnancy.

Conclusion

The key findings from this review that examined the benefits of providing specific nutrient supplements ranging from folic acid to LCPUFAs and even probiotics during pregnancy are summarized below.

(1) IFA supplements reduce the risk of anemia at term, but the evidence of reductions in the risks of LBW and PTD remains to be confirmed. Recent data suggest potential benefits that extend beyond birth especially in resource-poor settings. The benefits of IFA supplements in areas with endemic infection such as malaria have not been examined either.

(2) Multivitamin mineral supplements that provide 1–2 RDA of several key vitamins and minerals are safe during pregnancy and have the potential to reduce the burden of LBW in many developing countries where diets are suboptimal.

(3) Calcium supplementation can reduce the risk of preeclampsia and perhaps PTD in selected subgroups.

(4) Severe iodine deficiency has been associated with poor birth outcomes including severe mental retardation, but the benefits of iodine supplementation during pregnancy in mild to moderate iodine deficiency remain to be evaluated.

(5) Zinc supplementation can reduce the risk of PTD but not LBW. The optimal dosage and inclusion with other micronutrients needs more research.

(6) Prenatal LCPUFA supplementation may reduce the risk of PTD and improve cognitive performance. More studies, however, are needed to confirm the long-term benefits of prenatal LCPUFA supplementation.

(7) There is limited evidence to support the provision of supplements containing only vitamin A and D or antioxidants such as vitamins C and E. Existing data provide evidence of no benefits of providing antioxidants in reducing preeclampsia or PTD. Very few or no intervention trials have evaluated the independent effects of specific B vitamins such as vitamins B_6, B_{12} and folic acid on pregnancy outcomes, except for the protective effect of folic acid on NTDs during the periconceptual period.

(8) Probiotics can reduce genital infections, but the value of using them during pregnancy to improve child health remains to be evaluated.

Considerable progress has been made in our knowledge regarding the nature of nutrient interventions that can be recommended during pregnancy to optimize maternal and child health outcomes. Efforts to improve the preconceptual maternal nutritional status combined with timely and adequate access to antenatal care and providing interventions such as MMN supplements and minerals like calcium and zinc during pregnancy for at-risk populations would help promote the health and well-being of mothers and their offspring in a cost-effective manner. More research, however, is needed for interventions such as LCPUFAs and probiotics.

References

1 UNICEF: State of the Worlds Children 2009: Maternal and Newborn Health. New York, UNICEF, 2009.

2 Black RE, Allen LH, Bhutta ZA, Caulfield LE, de Onis M, Ezzati M, Mathers C, Rivera J: Maternal and child undernutrition: global and regional exposures and health consequences. Lancet 2008;371:243–260.

3 Bhutta ZA, Ahmed T, Black RE, Cousens S, Dewey K, Giugliani E, Haider BA, Kirkwood B, Morris SS, Sachdev HPS, Shekar M: What works? Interventions for maternal and child undernutrition and survival. Lancet 2008; 371:417–440.

4 Ramakrishnan U, Semba RD: Iron deficiency and anemia; in Semba RD, Bloem M (eds): Nutrition and Health in Developing Countries. Totawa, Humana Press, 2008, pp 479–505.

5 Centers for Disease Control: Recommendations to prevent and control iron deficiency in the United States. MMWR Recomm Rep 1998;47:1–29.

6 World Health Organization: Iron deficiency anemia: assessment, prevention and control. A guide for programme managers. 2001. http://www.who.int/nutrition/publications/micronutrients/anaemia_iron_deficiency/WHO_NHD_01.3/en/index.html.

7 Peña-Rosas JP, Viteri FE: Effects and safety of preventitive oral iron or iron + folic acid supplementation for women during pregnancy. Cochrane Database Syst Rev 2009; 7:CD004736.

8 World Health Organization: Weekly iron-folic supplementation (WIFS) in women of reproductive age: its role in promoting optimal maternal and child health (position statement). Geneva, WHO, 2009. http://www.who.int/nutrition/publications/micronutrients/weekly_iron_folicacid.pdf.

9 Zeng L, Cheng Y, Dang S, Yan H, Dibley MJ, Chang S, Kong L: Impact of micronutrient supplementation during pregnancy on birth weight, duration of gestation, and perinatal mortality in rural western China: double blind cluster randomised controlled trial. BMJ 2008;337:a2001.
10 Christian P, Khatry SK, Katz J, Pradhan EK, LeClerq SC, Shrestha SR, Adhikari RK, Sommer A, West KP Jr: Effects of alternative maternal micronutrient supplements on low birth weight in rural Nepal: double blind randomised community trial. BMJ 2003; 326:571.
11 Christian PS, Darmstadt GL, Wu L, Khatry SK, LeClerq SC, Katz J, West KP Jr, Adhikari RK: The impact of maternal micronutrient supplementation on early neonatal morbidity in rural Nepal: a randomized, controlled, community trial. Arch Dis Child Fetal Neonatal Ed 2007, Epub ahead of print.
12 Christian P, Stewart CP, LeClerq SC, Wu L, Katz J, West KP Jr, Khatry SK: Antenatal and postnatal iron supplementation and childhood mortality in rural Nepal: A prospective follow-up in a randomized, controlled community trial. Am J Epidemiol 2009;170: 1127–1136.
13 Wolff T, Witkop CT, Miller T, Syed SB: Folic acid supplementation for the prevention of neural tube defects: an update of the evidence for the US Preventive Services Task Force. Ann Intern Med 2009;150:632–639.
14 Centers for Disease Control: Spina bifida and anencephaly before and after folic acid mandate – United States, 1995–1996 and 1999–2000. MMWR Morb Mortal Wkly Rep 2004;53:362–365.
15 Haider BA, Bhutta ZA: Multiple-micronutrient supplementation for women during pregnancy. Cochrane Database of Sys Rev 2006;18:CD004905.
16 Ramakrishnan U, Gonzalez-Cossio T, Neufeld LM, Rivera J, Martorell R: Multiple micronutrient supplementation during pregnancy does not lead to greater infant birth size than does iron-only supplementation: a randomized controlled trial in a semirural community in Mexico. Am J Clin Nutr 2003; 77:720–725.
17 Roberfroid D, Huybregts L, Lanou H, Henry M-C, Meda N, Menten J, Kolsteren P, MSG: Effects of maternal multiple micronutrient supplementation on fetal growth: a double-blind randomized controlled trial in rural Burkina Faso. Am J Clin Nutr 2008;88:1330–1340.
18 Shankar A, Jahari A, Sebayang S, Aditiawarman, Apriatni M, Harefa B, Muadz H, Soesbandoro S, Tjiong R, Fachry A, Shankar A, Atmarita, Prihatini S, Sofia G: Effect of maternal multiple micronutrient supplementation on fetal loss and infant death in Indonesia: a double-blind cluster-randomised trial. Lancet 2008;371:215–227.
19 Zagre NM, Desplats G, Adou P, Mamadoultaibou A, Aguayo VM: Prenatal multiple micronutrient supplementation has greater impact on birth weight than supplementation with iron and folic acid: a cluster-randomized, double-blind, controlled programmatic study in rural Niger. Food Nutr Bull 2007; 28:317–327.
20 Fawzi W, Msamanga GI, Spiegelman D, Urassa EJN, McGrath N, Mwakagile D, Antelman G, Mbise R, Herrera G, Kapiga S, Willett W, Hunter DJ: Randomised trial of effects of vitamin supplements on pregnancy outcomes and T cell counts in HIV-1-infected women in Tanzania. Lancet 1998;351: 1477–1482.
21 Friis H, Gomo E, Nyazema N, Ndhlovu P, Krarup H, Kaestel P, Michaelsen KF: Effect of multimicronutrient supplementation on gestational length and birth size: a randomized, placebo-controlled, double-blind effectiveness trial in Zimbabwe. Am J Clin Nutr 2004;80:178–184.
22 Hininger I, Favier M, Arnaud J, Faure H, Thoulon JM, Hariveau E, Favier A, Roussel AM: Effects of a combined micronutrient supplementation on maternal biological status and newborn anthropometrics measurements: a randomized double-blind, placebo-controlled trial in apparently healthy pregnant women. Eur J Clin Nutr 2004;58: 52–59.
23 Kæstel P, Michaelsen KF, Aaby P, Friis H: Effects of prenatal multimicronutrient supplements on birth weight and perinatal mortality: a randomised, controlled trial in Guinea-Bissau. Eur J Clin Nutr 2005;59: 1081–1089.
24 Fawzi WW, Msamanga GI, Urassa W, Hertzmak E, Petraro P, Willett W, Spiegelman D: Vitamins and perinatal outcomes among HIV-negative women. N Engl J Med 2007; 356:1423–1441.
25 Gupta P, Ray M, Dua T, Radhakrishnan G, Kumar R, Sachdev HPS: Multimicronutrient supplementation for undernourished pregnant women and the birth size of their offspring: a double-blind, randomized, placebo-controlled trial. Arch Pediatr Adolesc Med 2007;161:58–64.
26 Osrin D, Vaidya A, Shrestha Y, Baniya RB, Manandhar DS, Adhikari RK, Filteau S, Tomkins A, de L Costello AM: Effects of antenatal multiple micronutrient supplementation on birth weight and gestational duration in Nepal: double-blind, randomised controlled trial. Lancet 2005;365:955–962.
27 Christian P, Osrin D, Manandhar DS, Khatry SK, de L Costello AM, West Jr KP: Antenatal micronutrient supplements in Nepal. Lancet 2005;366:711–712.
28 Shah PS, Ohlsson A: Effects of prenatal multimicronutrient supplementation on pregnancy outcomes: a meta-analysis. CMAJ 2009;180:E99–E108.
29 Hofmeyr G, Duley L, Atallah A: Dietary calcium supplementation for prevention of preeclampsia and related problems: a systematic review and commentary. BJOG 2007;114: 933–943.
30 Villar J, Abdel-Aleem H, Merialdi M, Mathai M, Ali MM, Zavaleta N, Purwar M, Hofmeyr J, Nhu Ngoc N, Campódonico L, Landoulsi S, Carroli G, Lindheimer M: World Health Organization randomized trial of calcium supplementation among low calcium intake pregnant women. Am J Obstet Gynecol 2006;194:639–649.
31 Kumar A, Devi SG, Batra S, Singh C, Shukla DK: Calcium supplementation for the prevention of pre-eclampsia. Int J Gynecol Obstet 2009;104:32–36.
32 Makrides M, Crowther CA: Magnesium supplementation in pregnancy. Cochrane Database Syst Rev 2001:CD000937.
33 Zimmermann MB: Iodine deficiency in pregnancy and the effects of maternal iodine supplementation on the offspring: a review. Am J Clin Nutr 2009;89:668S–672S.
34 West KP, Darnton-Hill I: Vitamin A deficiency; in Semba RD, Bloem MW (eds): Nutrition and Health in Developing Countries. Totowa, Humana Press, 2008, pp 377–433.
35 Kongnyuy EJ, Wiysonge CS, Shey MS: A systematic review of randomized controlled trials of prenatal and postnatal vitamin A supplementation of HIV-infected women. Int J Gynaecol Obstet 2009;104:5–8.
36 Coutsoudis A, Pillay K, Spooner E, Kuhn LA, Coovadia HM: Randomized trial testing the effect of vitamin A supplementation on pregnancy outcomes and early mother-to-child HIV-1 transmission in Durban, South Africa. AIDS 1999;13:1517–1524.
37 Fawzi W, Msamanga GIF, Hunter DAB, Renjifo BC, Antelman GA, Bang HB, Manji KG, Kapiga SD, Mwakagile DH, Essex MC, Spiegelman DBE: Randomized trial of vitamin supplements in relation to transmission of HIV-1 through breastfeeding and early child mortality. AIDS 2002;16:1935–1944.
38 Kumwenda N, Miotti PG, Taha TE, Broadhead R, Biggar RJ, Jackson JB, Melikian G, Semba RD: Antenatal vitamin A supplementation increases birth weight and decreases anemia among infants born to human immunodeficiency virus-infected women in Malawi. Clin Infect Dis 2002;35:618–624.
39 Humphrey JH, Iliff PJ, Marinda ET, Mutasa K, Moulton LH, Chidawanyika H, Ward BJ, Nathoo KJ, Malaba LC, Zijenah LS, Zvandasara P, Ntozini R, Mzengeza F, Mahomva AI, Ruff AJ, Mbizvo MT, Zunguza CD: Effects of a single large dose of vitamin A, given during the postpartum period to HIV-positive women and their infants, on child HIV infection, HIV-free survival, and mortality. J Infect Dis 2006;193:860–871.

40 Villamor E, Saathoff E, Bosch RJ, Hertzmark E, Baylin A, Manji K, Msamanga G, Hunter DJ, Fawzi WW: Vitamin supplementation of HIV-infected women improves postnatal child growth. Am J Clin Nutr 2005;81:880–888.
41 West KP Jr, Katz J, Khatry SK, LeClerq SC, Pradhan EK, Shrestha SR, Connor PB, Dali SM, Christian P, Pokhrel RP, Sommer A: Double blind, cluster randomised trial of low dose supplementation with vitamin A or β-carotene on mortality related to pregnancy in Nepal. BMJ 1999;318:570–575.
42 Hess SY, King JC: Effects of maternal zinc supplementation on pregnancy and lactation outcomes. Food Nutr Bull 2009;30:S60–S78.
43 Mahomed K, Bhutta Z, Middleton P: Zinc supplementation for improving pregnancy and infant outcome. Cochrane Database Syst Rev 2007;18:CD000230.
44 Zeyrek D, Soran M, Cakmak A, Kocyigit A, Iscan A: Serum copper and zinc levels in mothers and cord blood of their newborn infants with neural tube defects: a case-control study. Indian Pediatr 2009;46:675–680.
45 Erkkola M, Kaila M, Nwaru BI, Kronberg-Kippilä C, Ahonen S, Nevalainen J, Veijola R, Pekkanen J, Ilonen J, Simell O, Knip M, Virtanen SM: Maternal vitamin D intake during pregnancy is inversely associated with asthma and allergic rhinitis in 5-year-old children. Clin Exp Allergy 2009;39:875–882.
46 Rumbold A, Duley L, Crowther CA, Haslam RR: Antioxidants for preventing pre-eclampsia. Cochrane Database Syst Rev 2008; 23:CD004227.
47 Villar J, Purwar M, Merialdi M, Zavaleta N, Ngoc NTN, Anthony J, Greeff AD, Poston L, Shennan A: World Health Organisation multicentre randomised trial of supplementation with vitamins C and E among pregnant women at high risk for pre-eclampsia in populations of low nutritional status from developing countries. BJOG 2009;116:780–788.
48 Carlson SE: Docosahexaenoic acid supplementation in pregnancy and lactation. Am J Clin Nutr 2009;89:678S–684S.
49 Koletzko B, Lien E, Agostoni C, Bohles H, Campoy C, Cetin I, Decsi T, Dudenhausen JW, Dupont C, Forsyth S, Hoesli I, Holzgreve W, Lapillonne A, Putet G, Secher NJ, Symonds M, Szajewska H, Willatts P, Uauy R: The roles of long-chain polyunsaturated fatty acids in pregnancy, lactation and infancy: review of current knowledge and consensus recommendations. J Perinat Med 2008;36: 5–14.
50 Horvath A, Koletzko B, Szajewska H: Effect of supplementation of women in high-risk pregnancies with long-chain polyunsaturated fatty acids on pregnancy outcomes and growth measures at birth: a meta-analysis of randomized controlled trials. Br J Nutr 2007; 98:253–259.
51 Szajewska H, Horvath A, Koletzko B: Effect of n-3 long-chain polyunsaturated fatty acid supplementation of women with low-risk pregnancies on pregnancy outcomes and growth measures at birth: a meta-analysis of randomized controlled trials. Am J Clin Nutr 2006;83:1337–1344.
52 Krauss-Etschmann S, Shadid R, Campoy C, Hoster E, Demmelmair H, Jimenez M, Gil A, Rivero M, Veszpremi B, Decsi T, Koletzko BV, Nutrition and Health Lifestyle Study Group: Effects of fish-oil and folate supplementation of pregnant women on maternal and fetal plasma concentrations of docosahexaenoic acid and eicosapentaenoic acid: a European randomized multicenter trial. Am J Clin Nutr 2007;85:1392–1400.
53 Ramakrishnan U, Stein A, Parra-Cabrera S, Wang M, Imhoff-Kunsch B, Juarez-Marquez S, Rivera J, Martorell R: Effects of docosahexaenoic acid supplementation during pregnancy on gestational age and size at birth: randomized, double-blind, placebo-controlled trial in Mexico. Food Nutr Bull (in press).
54 Hibbeln JR, Davis JM, Steer C, Emmett P, Rogers I, Williams C, Golding J: Maternal seafood consumption in pregnancy and neurodevelopmental outcomes in childhood (ALSPAC study): an observational cohort study. Lancet 2007;369:578–585.
55 Helland IB, Smith L, Saarem K, Saugstad OD, Drevon CA: Maternal supplementation with very-long-chain n-3 fatty acids during pregnancy and lactation augments children's IQ at 4 years of age. Pediatrics 2003;111:e39–e44.
56 Dunstan JA, Simmer K, Dixon G, Prescott SL: Cognitive assessment of children at age 2 1/2 years after maternal fish oil supplementation in pregnancy: a randomised controlled trial. Arch Dis Child Fetal Neonatal Ed 2008;93:F45–F50.
57 Kopp MV, Salfeld P: Probiotics and prevention of allergic disease. Curr Opin Clin Nutr Metab Care 2009;12:298–303.
58 Kalliomäki M, Salminen S, Arvilommi H, Kero P, Koskinen P, Isolauri E: Probiotics in primary prevention of atopic disease: a randomised placebo-controlled trial. Lancet 2001;357:1076–1079.
59 Shadid R, Haarman M, Knol J, Theis W, Beermann C, Rjosk-Dendorfer D, Schendel DJ, Koletzko BV, Krauss-Etschmann S: Effects of galactooligosaccharide and long-chain fructooligosaccharide supplementation during pregnancy on maternal and neonatal microbiota and immunity: a randomized, double-blind, placebo-controlled study. Am J Clin Nutr 2007;86:1426–1437.
60 Othman M, Neilson JP, Alfirevic Z: Probiotics for preventing preterm labour (review). Cochrane Database Syst Rev 2007;24:-CD005941.